CHEMICAL WARFARE
AGENTS
TOXICOLOGY AND TREATMENT

CHEMICAL WARFARE AGENTS
TOXICOLOGY AND TREATMENT

Timothy C. Marrs
Department of Health, Skipton House, London, UK.

Robert L. Maynard
Department of Health, Skipton House, London, UK.

Frederick R. Sidell
US Army Medical Research Institute of Chemical Defense,
Aberdeen Proving Ground, Maryland, USA.

JOHN WILEY & SONS
Chichester · New York · Brisbane · Toronto Singapore

Copyright © 1996 by John Wiley & Sons Ltd,
Baffins Lane, Chichester,
West Sussex PO19 1UD, England

National   01243 779777
International   (+44) 1243 779777

Reprinted January 1997, April and December 1998, February 2000, June 2002.

Other Wiley Editorial Offices

John Wiley & Sons, Inc., 605 Third Avenue,
New York, NY 10158–0012, USA

Jacaranda Wiley Ltd, 33 Park Road, Milton,
Queensland 4064, Australia

John Wiley & Sons (Canada) Ltd, 22 Worcester Road,
Rexdale, Ontario M9W 1LI, Canada

John Wiley & Sons (Asia) Pte Ltd, 2 Clementi Loop #02-01,
Jin Xing Distripark, Singapore 05 12

Library of Congress Cataloging-in-Publication Data

Marrs, Timothy C.
    Chemical warfare agents : toxicology and treatment / Timothy C.
Marrs, Robert L. Maynard, Frederick R. Sidell.
        p.   cm.
    Includes bibliographical references and index.
    ISBN 0 471 95994 4 (alk. paper)
      1. Chemical agents (Munitions)—Toxicology.   2. Antidotes.
1. Maynard, Robert L. II. Sidell, Frederick R. III. Title.
RA64B.M37 1996
615.9—dc20   95-44142
                                                   CIP

British Library Cataloguing in Publication Data

A catalogue record for this book is available from the British Library

ISBN 0 471 95994 4

Typeset in 10/12pt Times by Techset Composition Ltd, Salisbury, Wiltshire
Printed and bound in Great Britain by Antony Rowe Ltd, Chippenham, Wiltshire
This book is printed on acid-free paper responsibly manufactured from sustainable forestation,
for which at least two trees are planted for each one used for paper production.

CONTENTS

PREFACE

Major advances have occurred in the last few years in our understanding of the mode of action of the classical chemical warfare agents and in their treatment. The collapse of the Soviet Union and of the Warsaw Pact led many people to expect a new era of goodwill between nations. However, events in the Gulf War have shown that developing countries may obtain the means to synthesize classical chemical warfare agents. It is therefore likely that future scenarios for chemical warfare may include small-scale or local conflicts where one or more parties are countries with a capacity to wage chemical warfare.

This book aims to cover the toxicology of the major groups of classical chemical warfare agents, including mechanisms of action, pathology and treatment of the resultant poisoning. Emphasis is placed upon the more practical aspects of treatment, including the particular difficulties of treatment in the field. The book will be of interest to all those in the chemical warfare field, including armed forces health care professionals, those engaged in civil defence planning and scientists working in the field. Some parts of the book will interest groups such as respiratory toxicologists. The chapters on organophosphate nerve agents may profitably be studied by those dealing with other types of organophosphorus compounds, such as those used as pesticides.

The book was partly written while two of the authors were working at the Chemical Defence Establishment (now the Chemical and Biological Defence Establishment), Porton Down, near Salisbury, in England. Our thanks are due to the Director, Dr Graham Pearson, and the Deputy Director (Biomedical), Dr Frank Beswick. Much of the work reported here was done at CBDE under the guidance and encouragement of these senior colleagues.

We would also like to acknowledge ex-colleagues, including Mr John Bright, Dr R. I. Gleadle, Dr M. C. French and Mr N. Cross, who, over a period of years, contributed to the development of many of the ideas expressed here. One of us (RLM) would also like to recognize the great assistance he has derived from the works of Dr Julian Perry Robinson and to thank him for his encouragement when this book was in an early stage of preparation. In addition we should like to thank Miss Julie Cumberlidge, who corrected many errors in the references quoted and helped order the final product.

It should be noted that the views expressed in this book are the personal ones of the authors and do not necessarily represent the views of any US or UK government departments.

1

OPINIONS OF CHEMICAL WARFARE

Chemical warfare should be abolished among nations, as abhorrent to civilisation. It is a cruel, unfair and improper use of science. It is fraught with the gravest danger to non-combatants and demoralises the better instincts of humanity.[1] Gen. Pershing

I claim, then, that the use of mustard gas in war on the largest possible scale would render it less expensive of life and property, shorter and more dependent upon brains than upon numbers.[2] Haldane

In no future war will the military be able to ignore poison gas. It is a higher form of killing.[3]

It is more difficult than might be supposed to say why poison gas seems to be such an immoral weapon to so many people.[4]

Chemical warfare (CW) has attracted opprobrium since it was first used on a large scale during World War I (WWI). Since 1919, efforts to persuade governments to abandon chemical weapons have been made by members of many sections of society—including the military—and yet, in the early 1990s, the number of countries believed to have, or to be procuring, the means to wage a chemical war is accepted to have never been higher. Third World countries, in particular, have become interested in chemical weaponry, and the use of such weapons by Iraq in the recent Iran–Iraq conflict attracted considerable Third World interest, yet disappointingly little and rather low-key censure from Western nations.

Over the past 74 years, chemical weapons have found only a few defenders. These have included such distinguished scientists as F. Haber and J. B. S. Haldane; military men, including Brigadier Fries and Lt. Col. Prentiss of the US Chemical Corps; military physicians, including Col. E. B. Vedder (US); and military historians, including B. H. Liddell Hart. Several of these writers had first-hand experience of the extensive use of chemicals during WWI, and despite, or perhaps because of, this advocated strongly the advantages and *humanity* of chemical weapons as compared with high explosives and fragmentation devices.

Such advocacy has had little effect, and the general repugnance for chemical weapons felt by the public and expressed by politicians and pressure groups has grown. During the late 1980s, fresh attempts to produce a ban on chemicals have been made. At the same time as these efforts have been underway, the threat of terrorists acquiring access to chemical weapons has increased.

As stated above, the general public and politicians have long reserved a special dislike and level of criticism for chemical weapons. CW devices are frequently referred to as immoral, cruel, inhumane, a debasement of science, unfair, etc. It is certainly true that many people hold such views. In enquiring into the origins of these views, writers have found difficulty in identifying precisely what it is about chemical weapons that people so dislike and disapprove of—as compared, of course, with other lethal weapon systems. The level of dislike encountered should not be underestimated: indeed, many more people in the UK probably disapprove of the use of CW by Germany during WWI than disapprove of the use of the much more destructive nuclear weapons by the USA during WWII. The roots of the disapproval are tangled and involve perceptions of where right lies in a conflict, of the use of particular weapons likely to hasten the end of the conflict, and a feeling that enemies who commit atrocities should be severely punished.

Of all the means of killing and waging war available to humankind, only biological warfare (BW) attracts more dislike and obloquy than CW. Notions of awful plagues spreading through the people of continents and possibly the world have been increased by popular authors and journalists, and little credence is given to anyone who argues that limited BW or even CW could be waged. Such opinions are seen as a form of warmongering, or of a descent into madness, and are vigorously opposed.

HISTORY OF CHEMICAL WARFARE

Throughout history, humans have sought more efficient means of killing their fellow humans. Stones, clubs, spears, arrows, gunpowder, muskets, rifles, high explosives, machine guns, tanks, warships, warplanes, rockets and nuclear weapons form an apparently unending catalogue of increasing military sophistication in destroying one's enemies, whilst exposing oneself, or the majority of one's forces, to decreasing risk. No means of stemming this tide of weapons has been discovered by accident and, until comparatively recent times, no efforts to find such means had been made. Accompanying this development of hardware, based on the production of physical disruption of people or materials, has been a much less marked development of chemical means of attacking people. Very little effort has been made to devise chemical means of attacking inanimate objects, and military smokes, and, more recently, infrared screening smokes, are the only significant examples of the use of chemicals to frustrate military equipment.

Chemical weapons probably began with smoke and flame. The lighting of bonfires and the hurling of various concoctions of pitch and sulphur (Greek Fire) date from classical times. Irritant smokes were described by Plutarch, hypnotics by the Scottish historian Buchanan, compounds capable of producing incessant diarrhoea by classical Greek authors,[5] and a whole range of preparations, including arsenical compounds and those containing the saliva of rabid dogs (a remarkably prescient notion), by Leonardo da Vinci.[6] During these remote periods, chemistry and chemical technology were in their infancy, and the use of chemical weapons probably had only a marginal effect on the outcome of wars. Such weapons would, perhaps, have had some terror-inducing effect rather along the lines of all secret weapons, possessed, or alleged to be possessed, by one force but not the other. These early examples of chemical weapons should be distinguished from the early use of poison as a means of removing small numbers of one's enemies. Poisoning probably dates from very earliest times, and Indian sources[5] from the fourth century BC reveal the use of alkaloids and toxins, including abrin (a compound closely related to ricin, the compound used to kill G. Markow in 1979). Aconite has a long history, and murderous Indian courtesans were reported to coat their lips with an impermeable substance and then apply aconite as a form of lipstick. One kiss, or probably several kisses and a bite, from such ladies was said to mean death. (Some sources allege the lethal dose of pure aconite to be as low as 7 mg.) Poisonous snakes and spiders have also been used as sources of strong poisons. Early 'researchers' in the old 'poison lore' recorded the effects of their preparations in detail, and the death of Britannicus (brother of Nero) is particularly well documented. Some practitioners undertook clinical experimental work, and Madame de Brinvilliers, who poisoned most of her relatives and developed powders known as 'Les poudres des succession', experimented upon hospital patients in Paris to assay the strengths and determine the effects of her preparations.[7] From the fifteenth to seventeenth centuries poisoning was rife in Italy, and it is probably from this period, when the postmortem detection of poisoning was all but impossible, that a deep dislike of poison, as a means of killing and achieving one's goals, stems. (It is also true to say that punishments for convicted poisoners at the time were particularly severe, boiling alive and the forced drinking of vast quantities of water being preferred methods.[7]) This condemnation of poisoning does not seem to have extended to the military use of chemicals before the nineteenth century, but suggestions that fumes of sulphur (sulphur dioxide) should be used as a weapon, made by Admiral Sir Thomas Cochrane (10th Earl of Sunderland) in 1855, were treated with disdain by the British military establishment.[5]

During WWI, chemicals were used on a vast scale: 12 000 tons of mustard gas alone, and, in all, 113 000 tons of chemicals were used.[8] Considerable attention has been paid to the identification of the first uses of CW during WWI and, therefore, the identity of the original transgressor of the Hague declarations of 1899 and 1907 (see below). It is likely that during the latter part of 1914, both Germany and France made use of non-lethal tear-gases, but on 22 April 1915 Germany launched a massive chlorine gas cloud attack, producing 15 000 Allied wounded and 5000 Allied dead. This attack came as a great surprise to the Allied governments, and not until 25 September 1915 could British forces launch their own chlorine cloud attacks. Phosgene was introduced by Germany late in 1915, and sulphur mustard on 12 July 1917.[8] Again, Allied governments were surprised, though scientists had advised of the likely military value of this compound, and not until September 1918 (two months before the Armistice) could British forces fire any mustard gas shells.

It is difficult to assess the military importance of CW during WWI. Enthusiasts for CW, e.g. Prentiss,[8] stressed the efficiency of the weapon, whereas other writers, including Fritz Haber's son,[9] pointed out that once adequate protective equipment became available, the efficacy and efficiency of CW fell sharply away.

During the period immediately following WWI, public opinion swung firmly against chemical warfare. Reasons for this are considered below. Minor uses of chemicals were alleged during the Russian Revolution (White Russian forces used British devices in 1919). Such weapons were also alleged to have been used by the Spanish in Morocco in 1925, and by Chinese forces in the early 1930s, but not until the Italian campaign in Ethiopia (1935–1936) were chemicals used again on a large scale: mustard gas was deployed with great effect against native Ethiopian troops.[1] Arguments regarding the ethics of such use are considered at length below.

During WWII, and despite, or perhaps because of, a great deal of civil defence effort (in the UK air raid precautions (ARP) were originally intended to defend against aerial gas attacks rather than attacks with high explosives), no proven incidents involving CW were reported in Europe. Japan did use CW against Chinese forces in the late 1930s and early 1940s. Reasons for the non-use of CW by Germany remain obscure but there can be no doubt of German superiority in the CW field: the development of so-called nerve gases tabun, sarin and soman in Germany between 1936 and 1944 came as an almost complete surprise to Allied scientists in 1945.[10] By 1945, some 12 000 tons of tabun had been made in Germany; none had been synthesized by Allied workers. Work on related compounds was certainly underway in the UK and the USA, but the breakthrough to nerve agents had not been made by these countries by 1945.

From 1945 until the 1980s, only two varieties of CW agents were used to any significant extent: lacrimators (CS: tear-gas) and herbicides (e.g. Agent Orange) by US forces in Vietnam. Allegations of CW use had been plentiful during the period and seem particularly convincing regarding Egyptian use of CW in the Yemen (1963–1967). During the 1980s, extensive use was made of mustard gas, and latterly nerve agent (probably tabun), by Iraqi forces during the Iran–Iraq conflict. In one incident at Halabja, some 5000 Iranians and Kurds were reported to have died as a result of a gas attack. Death on this scale, as a result of the use of CW, had not been known since the original German chlorine cloud attack of 1915.

Accusations of use of chemical weapons in South East Asia have been made and 'Yellow Rain' enjoyed a brief period of public attention. Despite intensive investigations, conclusive evidence of the deliberate use of trichothecene mycotoxins seems to be lacking. Allegations, rather better supported, of the use of CW by Soviet forces in Afghanistan have also been made, and a range of effects inexplicable in terms of known agents have been widely reported. Probably most recently, i.e. since 1985, allegations of the use of chemical weapons by Cuban or possibly other forces in Angola have been made, and, again, hard-to-explain effects have been reported. During 1988, reports of Libya constructing a chemical weapons production plant, and the publication in the March 1989 issue of the *Scientific American*[11] of what appears to be a satellite photograph of the plant, raised fears that terrorists might soon be able to acquire chemical weapons from sympathetic countries and a wave of new chemical terror might be unleashed.

These reported uses of CW and other matters have led to a general impression that whilst the superpowers may be approaching some measure of agreement regarding the undesirability of CW, Third World countries are not, and terrorists might well take up such weapons. Phrases such as 'the poor man's nuclear weapons' are often used in the press, and certainly a marked new interest in CW substances and how they might be produced has been generated.

THE PUBLIC PERCEPTION OF CW AND THE PERCEPTIONS OF NATIONAL LEADERS

It is difficult to separate the position of chemical weapons as regards international law from the public view of such devices. One might assume public opinion to be one of the forces which form international law, and it is probably true that international law, whether based on a treaty or upon alleged customary practice, would have little force unless it *were* supported by public opinion. Equally, public opinion, often based on poor information and very subject to propaganda, may be hardened and possibly formed by a well-publicized breach of international law. In the field of CW it is difficult to be definitive regarding the following question: does the illegality of CW depend upon treaties set up as a result of public opinion that CW is unethical, and therefore undesirable, or is the general public view that CW is unethical and presumably, therefore, undesirable, based upon the very existence of such treaties declaring this method of war illegal? An attempt to answer this question may be made by tracing the development of public opinion and international law regarding CW and attempting to separate examples of political expediency from military desires and ethical thinking. This will be followed by a closer examination of the role of ethical thinking in forming international law regarding CW and particularly of how the concept of the 'just war' has been applied to the topic.

As said already, CW has a long, if patchy, history and was waged on a large scale for the first time during WWI. It is, therefore, remarkable that efforts to prevent the use of chemicals in warfare were made *before*, albeit not very long before, WWI. The first Hague Conference held in 1899 formulated a resolution stating 'The Contracting Powers agree to abstain from the use of all projectiles, the sole object of which is the diffusion of asphyxiating or deleterious gases.' The precise wording regarding 'sole object ... ' resulted from an observation that all high explosive (HE) shells tended to generate noxious gases in some quantity and that such gases, in confined spaces, could be dangerous. The exact wording was later used by Germany to justify her use of shells containing shrapnel balls embedded in an irritant chemical powder, on 27 October 1914, on the grounds that the diffusion of asphyxiating or deleterious gases was not the *sole* purpose of such munitions.

Whilst the proposition received general assent, the USA stood out against it, and a statement by the Naval Delegate (Captain A. H. Mahan) expressed clearly a view that CW could not be regarded as an unusually appalling method of waging war. He said:

> It was illogical and not demonstrably humane, to be tender about asphyxiating men with gas, when all are prepared to admit that it was allowable to blow the bottom out of an ironclad at midnight, throwing four or five hundred men into the sea to be choked by water, with scarcely the remotest chance of escape.[12]

This particularly objective remark has remained the basis of thinking of those who have advanced the case of CW during the twentieth century. The problem of CW was, however, remote in 1899, and comparatively little attention was paid to the US position.

The Second Hague Conference of 1907 attempted to codify what were regarded as a number of unwritten rules of warfare, though CW, in the modern sense, was not considered. Article XXIII of the 1907 Hague Convention regarding Laws and Customs of War on Land deals with a closely related issue: 'In addition to the prohibitions provided by special conventions, it is especially forbidden to employ poison or poisoned weapons.' The USA clarified its position on poison and poisoned weapons in The Rules of Land Warfare, War Department Document No. 468, paragraph 177, wherein it was made clear that 'poison' applied to the contamination of water sources and the depositing therein of the carcases of animals. This codification by the USA represented an easing of the position adopted by that country in 1863 (General Orders War Department No. 100): 'The use of poison in any manner, be it to poison wells or food or arms, is wholly excluded from modern warfare.' It might be deduced from these several US statements that little conviction existed amongst the US senior military staff regarding the unethical nature of CW— they were, in fact, attempting to 'keep their options open'.

Such a deduction is supported by a US State Department opinion given at the time of the First Hague Conference:

> The expediency of restraining the inventive genius of our people in the direction of devising means of defense is by no means clear, and considering the temptations to which men and nations may be exposed in time of conflict, it is doubtful if an international agreement to this end would prove effective.[13]

In terms of the formation of international law regarding CW, the USA may be seen as opposing the formation of *conventional* law when no *customary* law existed.

The UK view in the pre-WWI period seems to have been much more clearly against the use of CW. This view was advanced most strongly in traditional military circles, and the suggestion, made in 1855 by Sir Thomas Cochrane, that fumes of burning sulphur should be used were met with the comment from the War Ministry that 'an operation of this nature would contravene the laws of a civilized warfare'.[1] The USA's refusal to adhere to the 1899 Hague Declaration meant that unanimity at the conference, a requirement of UK agreement, was impossible, and the UK did not so agree. In 1907, the UK did 'adhere to the declaration' and became bound by it. France agreed with the 1899 Hague Declaration, as did Germany, Italy, Russia and Japan.

The use of chlorine gas on a large scale by the Germans in 1915 took Allied forces and governments by surprise and a vigorous propaganda campaign deploring the use of such means of waging war was put in hand in the UK. This campaign, supported by lurid reports in the national press, mobilized public opinion against the German use of chemical weapons. Julian Perry Robinson[14] has studied the propaganda disseminated during the period following the German use of chlorine in detail, and has drawn attention to the following description of gas casualties from *The Times* of 30 April 1915, 'The Full Story of Ypres: a New German Weapon' (described as being contributed by 'an authority beyond question'), as revealing the approach taken:

> Their faces, arms, hands were of a shiny grey-black colour, with mouths open and lead glazed eyes, all swaying slightly backwards and forwards trying to get breath. It was a most appalling sight all those poor black faces, struggling, struggling for life what with the groaning and noise of the effort for breath. .... The effect the gas has is to fill the lungs with a watery frothy matter, which gradually increases and rises till it fills up the whole lungs and comes up to the mouth; then they die; it is suffocation; slow drowning, taking in some cases one or two days.

Germany responded with propaganda of the opposite kind:

> These shells* are not more deadly than the poison of the English explosives,† but they take effect over a wider area, produce a rapid end, and spare the torn bodies the tortures of pain and death.

Despite the launching of a propaganda attack on the German use of chlorine, the British government failed to protest vigorously that Germans had breached at least the spirit, if not the words, of the Hague Declaration of 1899. Protests were made when, later, Germany made use of chemical-containing shells. The British government was faced in 1915 by a very difficult problem: there was no doubt that general opinion was against the use of chemical weapons, but such weapons were clearly effective (15 000 wounded, 5000 dead and widespread panic induced during the first German gas attack) and seen by some as a means of breaking the deadlock of trench warfare. The British government took the view that, unfortunately

---

* The date of this quotation is 29 April 1915: 'Through German Eyes: poisonous gases: a quick and painless death' (*The Times*). Interestingly, at this time, no 'shells' had been used, and the German government was arguing that their use of gas clouds produced from cylinders and *not by shells* did not infringe the Hague Declaration of 1899.
† Refers to fumes produced on explosion of Lyddite, a picric-acid-based explosive.

and against its better instincts, chemicals would have to be used by British forces and began the manufacture of such weapons. Senior British military opinion remained firmly against chemical weapons: Sir John French (12 July 1915), referring to the German use of gas:

> As a soldier, I cannot help expressing the deepest regret and some surprise that an Army which, hitherto, has claimed to be the chief exponent of the chivalry of war, should have stooped to employ such devices against brave and gallant foes ....[15]

British opinion, then, was generally against the German use of chemicals, but accepted that as such weapons had been used and were seen to be effective, Britain would have no option but to reply in kind. The use of gas by British forces was at first represented as a reprisal against the German use of gas. However, gas use soon escalated and British use far passed any reasonable definition of a reprisal. By the close of WWI, CW seems to have been accepted as a regrettable fact of military life, and the existence of customary law against its use would have been difficult to demonstrate.

The US government responded more radically than had the British government when American troops suffered badly from chemical attacks during the early days after their entry into WWI. A Chemical Warfare Service (CWS) was set up and, with eventually 4873 men under the command of 210 officers, formed a force more committed to CW than any in the British Army. At the end of WWI, the CWS was markedly reduced and all but abolished; however, a vigorous and effective propaganda campaign ensured its survival. Articles published in chemical journals extolled the efforts of the CWS, and one editorial closed:

> Bestir yourselves, chemists of America! The country glories in the services you have already rendered it in peace and war. Opportunity for further service now presents itself. Whether we will it or not, gas will determine peace or victory in future wars. The Nation must be fully prepared![16]

DEVELOPMENT OF PUBLIC OPINION AFTER WWI

After WWI, public opinion regarding chemical weapons was influenced by a number of factors which may be worth considering briefly.

The general revulsion concerning war which followed WWI—the 'war to end war'—was marked, and triggered a pacifist movement which remained active during the period 1926–1934. CW had been the subject of much official propaganda during WWI and was seen by activists in the pacifist movements as the very embodiment of all that was evil about modern war. The view was driven deeply into the public mind by the work of several of the 'War Poets', who painted an awful picture of men dying of the effects of chlorine and being blinded by mustard gas. The efforts of the League of Nations and the holding of a series of conferences and meetings were based upon these general feelings that if warfare was evil, then CW was particularly evil. The feelings of revulsion described above were fuelled by post-war propaganda designed not only to remind people of the horrors of CW, but also to point out the alleged likely greater horrors if further development of this type of warfare were to be allowed. It should be said that such revelations came from several sources, one being the American CWS. Anxious to preserve its existence, the CWS undertook a series of what would be today regarded as 'leaks' designed to alert the public to the dangers of new chemical 'super-weapons'.

Chlorovinyl dichlorarsine, or lewisite, was often the subject of these disclosures, and this compound acquired a particularly bad reputation. Claims that this compound—'The Dew of Death'—was 'invisible', that if inhaled it 'killed at once', that 'three drops upon the skin would kill', and that the compound 'falling like rain from nozzles attached to an aeroplane, [it could] kill practically everyone in an area over which the aircraft passed' were made.[8,17,18] This theme was adopted by popular authors and 'Sapper' (pseudonym of Herman Cyril McNeil (1888–1937)) dwelt at length upon CW and lewisite in several of his anti-Bolshevik and anti-German 'Bulldog Drummond' romances. In Britain, a more cautious line was generally taken by supporters of the need for further work on CW, but, in an attempt to raise interest and support the work, the President of the Society of the Chemical Industry described a new CW agent against which gas masks offered no protection and which would 'stop a man' at a concentration of one in five million. 'Stop a man' is an emotive and imprecise phrase. To many people the phrase would suggest a lethal effect, though in the case of the compound being considered (Adamsite) severe lacrimation would be a much more likely response.

These efforts were supported vigorously by the Allied chemical industries, which, in retrospect, cannot but have been eager for their expansion and the destruction of the world's leading chemical industry: that of Germany. The extent of the German domination of the world chemical industry prior to WWI is often not appreciated. In 1913, Germany produced 85.91% of the world's dyes. Britain produced 2.54% and the USA 1.84%.[8] The six great German chemical firms had banded together prior to WWI to form Interessen Gemeinschaft Farben (IG Farben: community of interests: dyes) and completely dominated the production of organic chemicals. Fritz Haber, the chemist who organized the German use of chemicals during WWI, was closely associated with IG Farben; Schrader, the developer of nerve agents in the late 1930s, was later one of its leading chemists. British and American writers saw IG Farben, as others saw the Krupps armaments empire, as a dangerous threat and made efforts to have it dismantled and Allied industries expanded in its stead. This line of argument was most effectively pursued by Victor Lefebure in his book *The Riddle of the Rhine*.[19] Lefebure's arguments have been examined by more recent writers, and despite pointing out that he may have had some vested interest in seeing the decline of IG Farben (he was an employee of Imperial Chemical Industries), most agree that his was a good case, well argued. The line taken by commentators such as Lefebure in the UK and Vedder and others in the USA was not a pacifist one: they accepted CW as a likely fact of war and wished to ensure that neither the USA nor the UK should be found again at so great a disadvantage as they had been at the time of the first large-scale German CW attack in 1915.

In addition to those pointing out the horrors of CW was a small group of scientists and others who supported further work on CW for quite a different reason: they thought it was a *more* humane way to wage war than conventional means. The leading proponent of this view was J. B. S. Haldane, who had had first-hand experience of gas warfare as an officer in the Black Watch recalled from France to assist his father Professor J. S. Haldane (brother of Viscount Haldane) in undertaking research in CW. J. B. S. Haldane was frequently exposed to chlorine gas and various lacrimators and irritants. In 1925, he published a series of lectures on CW as a book entitled *Callinicus: A Defence of Chemical Warfare*.[2] (Haldane chose the title of the book in honour of the Syrian Callinicus, the alleged inventor of a pitch-tar and sulphur mixture called 'Greek Fire'. In his preface he pointed out that 'Callinicus' means 'He who conquers in a noble or beautiful manner'!) Referring to the lack of understanding of CW on the part of army officers:

> The chemical and physiological ideas which underlie gas warfare require a certain effort to understand, and they do not arise in the study of sport as is the case with those undertaking shooting and motor transport.

These attacks, combined with Haldane's growing, and carefully cultivated, reputation as an iconoclast, led to his opinions being widely disregarded.

Of medical officers involved in treating CW casualties, most stressed the very unpleasant nature of the effects of these weapons whilst not comparing them with injuries produced by other weapons systems. Many reports and papers in medical journals stressed the seriousness of mustard gas burns, though hardly any compared these burns with commonplace thermal burns. A few distinguished medical writers, again with extensive first-hand experience of CW, *did* publish comparative material but this also was largely ignored. Of these authors, Lt. Col. E. B. Vedder[20] is probably the best known. His book remains an indispensable and accurate account of those aspects of CW of interest to the physician. In Vedder's introduction, he acknowledges the 'considerable prejudice against the use of gas in warfare' and identifies three reasons for this prejudice:

1. That the Germans had used it first and were considered by many to have violated the Hague Declarations.
2. That it was a new weapon and all new weapons seemed to be instinctively disliked.
3. That CW was seen as barbarous and inhumane.

How such comments were received is difficult to establish some 70 years later: they did not, however, seem to convince many that CW was a new and inherently *more* acceptable form of warfare. It is also possible that by drawing attention to CW, public revulsion was increased.

There was then, after WWI, a preponderance of opinion in favour of the view that CW was a particularly unpleasant form of warfare and that those who supported it, with the exception of industrialists perceived to be concerned with preserving national security, were either cranks or simply deluded. These general feelings were reflected by the attempt by the USA to place some limits on the development of a variety of weapon systems by calling the Washington Conference on the Limitation of Armaments in 1921–1922. CW was referred to a subcommittee which considered the development of this form of warfare during WWI and concluded that it was impracticable to attempt to limit the use of chemicals any more than that of explosives, and stated, regarding chemical weapons: 'there can be no limitation on their use against the armed forces of the enemy, ashore or afloat'.[21] As Perry Robinson has pointed out, this view was in accord with the negotiating position of the US delegation.[14] However, when this was discussed at the conference, the US delegation strongly opposed the subcommittee report. This reversal of position seems to have been the result of intense lobbying and the activities of an advisory subcommittee to the US delegation which had been formed by C. E. Hughes, a US Senator. This group reported that:

> The frightful consequences of the use of toxic gases, if dropped from airplanes on cities, stagger the imagination .... If lethal gases were used in ... bombs (of the size used against cities in the war), it might well be that such permanent and serious damage would be done ... in the depopulation of large sections of the country as to threaten, if not destroy, all that has been granted during the painful centuries of the past.

The ludicrous nature of this assertion, given the level of technology available in 1921, need not be laboured, though it may be that members of the advisory subcommittee were more concerned about possible, though unlikely, future developments than the current position. The view of the advisory subcommittee was supported by a public opinion poll taken in the USA: 366 975 people wanted abolition; 19 wanted retention under the terms of the recommendations of the original subcommittee. The advice of the original subcommittee was rejected, the advice of the advisory subcommittee accepted, and the treaty ratified by most nations, including the USA and UK. France did not ratify the treaty, though not for any reasons of disagreement regarding CW, but rather for some regarding submarine warfare.[22]

By 1922, there seemed to exist a widespread consensus that CW was an especially undesirable form of warfare and one which should be prohibited by international convention. This desire to prohibit by treaty had been interpreted by some jurists as evidence of a perceived *lack* of any customary law prohibiting the use of chemical weapons.

The general enthusiasm for prohibition of CW was followed by the signing of the Geneva Protocol.[23] This protocol called for an acceptance of earlier conventions regarding CW and extended them to include bacteriological warfare. The wording regarding chemicals, taken from the 1922 Washington Treaty, prohibiting the use of 'Asphyxiating, poisonous or other gases, and all analogous liquids, materials or devices', was particularly wide-ranging and could be interpreted as embracing tear-gases, herbicides, incapacitants and other non-lethal compounds. As written, the protocol was a very clear reflection of public and national perceptions regarding CW in the 1920s. In the UK the Geneva Protocol was largely accepted by the military community; in the USA it was not, and intense pressure was brought to bear on the Senate Committee on Foreign Relations. The CWS and the US chemical industry orchestrated this pressure, and by December 1926 had so persuaded the Senate Committee on Military Affairs that the Chairman said:

> I think it is fair to say that in 1922, there was much of hysteria and much of misinformation concerning chemical warfare. I was not at all surprised at the time that the public generally—not only in this country but in many other countries—believed that something should be done to prohibit the use of gas in warfare. The effects of that weapon had not been studied at the time to such an extent to permit information about it to reach the public. There were many misconceptions as to its effects and as to the character of warfare involved in its use.[14]

The results of a survey of 3500 American physicians were quoted, demonstrating that there was an informed consensus that, in comparison with more conventional weapons, gas caused less suffering, both during exposure and during its after-effects. This view was supported by: The Association of Military Surgeons, The American Legion, The Veterans of Foreign Wars of the United States, the Reserve Officers Association of the United States and the Military Order of the World War.[14] This pressure was irresistible and the USA delayed ratification of the Geneva Protocol until 1975—and then agreed with reservations. Other countries also delayed ratification: UK, 1930; Germany, 1929; Ethiopia, 1935; and the USSR, 1928. France ratified the protocol in 1926. Many of those ratifying entered reservations, usually including the following:

1. The protocol could only be regarded as binding as regards states which had signed, ratified or acceded to it.
2. The protocol would *ipso facto* cease to be binding regarding a state failing to adhere to it.

These reservations seem like examples of simple common sense or prudence, but have been interpreted by some jurists as implying a lack of conviction amongst the contracting parties as regards the 'unthinkability' of CW in that they allow for the possibility of waging CW under certain circumstances.

During the period following the agreement (though not ratification) of the Geneva Protocol, public opinion, in general, remained against chemical weapons as a means of waging war. The International Committee of the Red Cross (ICRC) conferences held in the late 1920s agreed resolutions deploring CW. The ICRC also attempted to encourage work in the field of civil defence against CW and pointed out that the level of protection available to the public in many countries was lamentably low. In 1929, *The Times* reported the ICRC as offering a prize for the best mustard gas detector and of planning competitions for design of civilian anti-gas equipment.[23] One of the few countries to take such advice seriously was the USSR, and in 1928 a simulated

CW attack by 30 aeroplanes on Leningrad was undertaken. *The Times* reported a comment from *Izvestia* to the effect that the public regarded the powder bombs as more 'an ordinary street sight' than a 'serious exercise'![24] The public perception that gas attacks were so horrible to contemplate that no civilized country would indulge in such attack was widespread at this time.

In 1935–1936 this perception changed. Italian forces used mustard gas against Ethiopian troops to considerable effect. The Italians argued for their legitimate use of a weapon prohibited by international law in terms of its use being by way of a reprisal (and therefore seen as exempt from the usual requirements of international law) for the behaviour of Ethiopian troops in torturing and mutilating prisoners of war. This defence, or justification, of the use of CW was seen by the Italian government as acceptable, despite the fact that Italy had signed the Geneva Protocol in 1925 and ratified it in 1928. Interestingly, though, Italy had not entered the common reservations regarding the treaty ceasing to be binding under certain conditions and relied on the *customary* international law that reprisals may involve the use of means normally regarded as illegal. The maximum extent of such reprisals has never been specified, but it seems certain that Italy exceeded the spirit of the rules of war concerning such reprisals. It was noted in the UK and the USA that a fascist country, Italy, had used chemical weapons. Evidence was accumulating that Germany, under Hitler, was becoming interested both in chemical weapons and in strategic bombing as means of waging war. Wickham Steed wrote pointing out the dangers of German developments in these directions and stressed the dangers of 'aerochemical attacks on civilians'.[25] Efforts followed, in the UK, to develop air raid precautions against such attacks, and the *Air Raid Precautions Handbook No. 1*, published in 1936, was subtitled 'Personal Protection against Gas'.[26] Calculations undertaken by the UK and elsewhere revealed that CW attacks on civilians in cities were, in fact, not likely to be particularly effective: HE and, particularly, incendiary bombing was calculated to be likely to be very much more effective. However, ARP measures turned on the dangers of a gas attack, and by 1939 only babies in the UK had not been issued with respirators. The dangers of a CW attack were emphasized, though in a 'we can cope if we are careful' way designed not to induce panic, and measures for dealing with HE bombing were taught at the same time.

Public opinion before WWII was firmly against the use of chemical weapons, though it is clear that some national leaders took a different view, and Winston Churchill returned to his long-held belief in the merits of CW in a series of wartime statements—mainly not intended for public consumption. In 1940, Churchill asked for an assessment of the value of mustard gas as an anti-invasion measure, and by 1944 his view had become characteristically clear:

It may be several weeks or even months before I shall ask you to drench Germany with poison gas, and if we do it, let us do it one hundred per cent. In the meanwhile, I want the matter to be studied in cold blood by sensible people and not by that particular set of psalm-singing uninformed defeatists which one runs across now here, now there.[27]

It seems clear from this and remarks made earlier in his career that Churchill was prepared to contemplate the use of CW in what he saw as a just cause. The discovery of the very toxic nerve agents by Schrader in Germany just before and during WWII was a major surprise, as already stated, to the Allied powers, and the acquisition by the Soviet Union of the major German nerve agent production plants at Dühernfurt on the river Oder, now Dyhernfurth, Silesia, Poland, immediately after WWII, was seen as a particularly sinister development. The Soviet Union was understood to have acquired the technology to produce nerve agents in considerable quantities, and programmes of aggressive CW research were put in hand in both the USA and the UK. In the UK, an offensive, as compared with a defensive, policy of research and development in the CW field was abandoned in 1956. The reasons for this abandonment are difficult to establish, as many documents relating to the decision remain unavailable.

US policy has changed over the period: chemical weapons were produced until 1969.[28] President Nixon, in 1974, agreed with Secretary Brezhnev of the Soviet Union to consider a joint initiative on the prohibition of chemical weapons. This was confirmed by President Ford in 1976, and bilateral negotiations began in Geneva in that year. As after WWI, the US Chemical Army Corps (which replaced the CWS) was reduced in strength (from about 4000 to about 2000) and, as before, began a campaign of lobbying. This, combined with the concept of putting pressure on the Soviet Union by *improving* US weapons at the same time as arguing for their bilateral removal, led in 1981 to President Reagan permitting the production of so-called binary weapons. This programme has been subject to considerable criticism both inside the USA and within other NATO countries. In particular, attempts to store chemical weapons in Europe certainly met strong opposition. During the 1970s and early 1980s, public opinion regarding CW underwent little change. The proponents of CW argued for possession of weapons on the grounds that strong defence was vital and that the Soviet Union's pronouncements regarding its desire to abandon a capacity to conduct a chemical war should not be trusted. The opponents of CW have continued to argue that the use of such weapons would be reprehensible and their possession inevitably increased the likelihood of their use. Very little debate regarding the ethical aspects of CW took place during this period and articles arguing in favour of CW such as that by Liddell Hart, are scarce.[29] The view espoused by Haldane that CW was a good deal *more* desirable than conventional war seemed to have gone into eclipse.

Public opinion regarding CW changed little during the Iran–Iraq conflict in the 1980s, and standard condemnations of the use of chemical weapons were made by Western political leaders. These condemnations reveal no new thinking on, or rethinking of, the ethical aspects of CW but followed the usual assumption of the undesirability of CW and pointed out that it was prohibited under the terms of the Geneva Protocol of 1925. Iraq, the main user of CW during the conflict, had ratified the Geneva Protocol in 1931.

In summary, then, public opinion regarding CW seems to have been formed in the years following WWI. It was markedly influenced by propaganda regarding the peculiar unpleasantness of this type of warfare, spread both by those anxious to build up a national CW capability and those anxious to achieve a prohibition of the future use of chemical weapons. Though others argued in favour of CW, they seem to have had little influence and public opinion remains against these weapons.

CHEMICAL WARFARE EXAMINED FROM THE STANDPOINT OF THE CUSTOMARY RULES OF WAR

It is widely accepted by civilized nations that war should only be engaged in to achieve certain acceptable ends. Perceptions as to what comprise acceptable ends have changed in the course of history, and, for a long period, the expansion of one's state was seen as a perfectly acceptable purpose, with rulers engaging in wars to acquire more land or certain facilities, e.g. access to coasts, to water supplies, to better farmlands. Such reasons for going to war would not be seen as acceptable today. The opinion that wars should not be fought for reasons of expediency is embodied in the first of the often-quoted seven conditions which need to be satisfied before a war can be regarded as a *just war*.[30]

1. The war must be declared by the legitimate public authority and the action must aim at universal good; it must not be a matter of expediency.
2. The seriousness of the injury to be suffered [should war not be declared] must be proportional to the damages war will cause.
3. The seriousness of the injury to be suffered at the hands of the aggressor must be real and immediate.
4. There must be a reasonable chance of winning the war.
5. War may be initiated only as a last resort to redressing grievances.
6. A war may be prosecuted legitimately only insofar as the responsible agents have a right intention.
7. The particular means employed to wage the war must themselves be moral.

Points 1–6 refer to the *ius ad bellum*: the necessity of a just cause for a just war. Point 7 refers to the *ius in bello*: the necessity of just means of fighting for a just war.

The seven conditions have also been defined by J. J. Haldane[31]* in rather simpler terms:

1. The war must be made by a lawful authority.
2. The war must be waged for a morally just cause, e.g. self-defence.
3. The warring state must have a rightful intention, i.e. to pursue the just cause.
4. The war must be the only means of achieving the just end.
5. There must be a reasonable prospect of victory.
6. The good to be achieved must be greater than the probable evil effects of waging war.

---

* J. J. Haldane is currently senior lecturer in Moral Philosophy at St Andrews and should not be confused with Professor J. S. Haldane (1860–1936), who undertook research on CW during WWI with his son, Professor J. B. S. Haldane (1892–1964).

7. The means of war must not themselves be evil: either by being such as to cause gratuitous injuries or deaths, or by involving the intentional killing of innocent civilians.

Before considering the ethical aspects of CW in more detail, it may be as well to define three terms sometimes used in discussing this question:

Ethics   There are a number of definitions of ethics. The Shorter Oxford English Dictionary (SOD) defines 'ethics' as: 'the, or a, science of morals'. This definition and those like it have led many to confuse ethics with morals or ethical behaviour with moral behaviour. Russell[32] attempted to separate ethics from morals by defining ethically correct behaviour as transcending the requirements of any particular religious doctrine; for example, ethical behaviour could be defined as behaviour designed to increase the level of happiness of people.

Morals   Morals, or more easily moral codes, are considerably easier to understand than ethics or ethical codes. A moral code applies to behaviour and not to objects. In the Christian faith, basic moral standards of behaviour are laid down in the decalogue: 'Thou shalt not kill' etc. Moral teaching lays down rules of behaviour, for use in fairly specific cases.

Casuistry   Casuistry is the science of determining, on an ethical or moral basis, the correct action an individual should take under a given set of circumstances. As Russell has pointed out, casuistry has acquired a bad reputation and is sometimes seen as a branch of, or analogous to, sophistry. Casuistry attempts to define ethically and morally correct actions under a given set of circumstances, whereas sophistry is 'the use or practice of specious reasoning as an art of dialectic exercise' (SOD). Casuistry led to the very precise, but often probably pointless, arguments of medieval philosophers, and was often regarded as a destructive technique: 'Casuistry destroys, by distinctions and exceptions all morality' (Bolingbroke (SOD)). Unfortunately, condition 7 of the just war code requires a casuistic approach, and it will be demonstrated below that, on some occasions, to wage CW might be an ethically and morally correct act, but under other circumstances it might not.

An example of the difficulty encountered in applying an ethically and morally correct approach in war is provided by the case of the spy in time of war. Spying is held to be prohibited by generally accepted rules of war as unethical, and yet all countries capable of so doing engage in spying in peacetime and to such an extent as is possible in wartime. For a country perceived to be fighting a *just war*, it is difficult to regard the activities of its spies as unethical or immoral; of course, it is likely that the other country involved would also perceive its actions as just and have the same difficulty regarding its spies.

The importance of defining morally acceptable behaviour in terms of specific religious philosophies should not be overlooked. Different religions define different morally acceptable codes of conduct, and one cannot argue that use of a chemical weapon by an enemy is morally wrong unless the enemy subscribes to one's own religious beliefs and one has demonstrated that those beliefs lead to such use being held to be immoral. The difference between ethics and morals arises at this point.

One might hold an act by an enemy to be unethical though not immoral. The assumption here is that an ethical code which transcends all religious or moral codes could, in principle at least, be defined.

Ethical and moral thinking is often seen as leading to the definition of legal principles. Some have attempted to distinguish between the results of ethical and legal thinking, and J. J. Haldane[33] has defined the difference between legal principles and objective moral (he uses 'objective moral' and 'ethical' interchangeably) principles as:

> Law issues from the will of legislators, and binds those who fall within its scope either by knowingly consenting to be bound by it or else by acting in ways which imply their implicit acceptance of the rules of society. Morality, if it is objective, has a foundation independent of the human will and has a logically different kind of force upon us. What has been willed [i.e. a legal principle] can be opposed and revoked; what is the objective moral case, apart from human attitudes to it, remains such, however much as one or all may wish it were not so.

The critical difference between legal and ethical principles controls the way in which activities may be construed. By observing patterns of activity one can arrive at a 'descriptive norm' of behaviour. This is an adequate basis for a legal principle. On the other hand, observing how people act is logically of no value whatsoever in defining how they *should* act, i.e. in defining a norm of behaviour *prescriptively*. Knowing that Germany and Britain used CW during WWI and that Germany and Britain did not use CW during WWII is of no assistance in defining how they *should* have behaved or how they *should* behave in the future. Defining an ethically acceptable pattern of behaviour is very much more difficult than defining a legally acceptable one; though if it can be done it will likely last longer and likely be more effective. J. J. Haldane has said in considering the establishment of constraints on the use of biological (though his argument applies with equal force to chemical) weapons, 'only morality *could* provide an inescapable external constraint'.

Some authorities, including Sims,[34] have been concerned about the origins of attitudes and beliefs regarding chemical, biological and nuclear warfare. It has often been said (see above) that revulsion regarding CW is an instinctive response. Such responses are generally seen as automatic, dependent upon genetic factors and cultural patterns and as independent of reason. On the other hand, it has been held that a prerequisite for a satisfactory ethical or moral belief is that it should be based upon a rational and demonstrably true judgement. Given that instinctive responses may not necessarily be rationally based, it has been argued that an ethical judgement founded upon an instinctive belief is unsatisfactory and may be unconvincing. J. J. Haldane has considered the following question (my paraphrasing) as regards BW, though the thrust of his answer applies equally to CW: Does the possibility of one's revulsion from induced plague being an instinctive response exclude it from being a moral judgement? He commented:

> This line of thought instantiates the fallacy of supposing that if one has a 'genetic' explanation of why someone is in a certain psychological state, e.g. because of their nature or upbringing, the question of the rationality or truth does not arise. This is fallacious because the origin of a belief is logically independent of its content. Thus, whether an expression of revulsion is instinctive or the product of reflection does not touch upon the issue of whether it is a genuine moral judgement, or whether, if it is such, it is justified and true. These questions can only be answered by looking at the content of the expression.

This is a most important comment and one which strikes in two directions.

The view that CW is unethical *by virtue* of the widespread instinctive revulsion it engenders is dismissed, as is the concern that an ethical judgement based upon such an instinctive revulsion is inevitably flawed. One might conclude that the existence of a marked instinctive revulsion regarding CW is of no relevance in assessing the ethical or moral propriety of this form of warfare.

Certain standards of acceptable behaviour can be defined, indeed have been defined, and comprise the basis of the generally accepted rules of conduct of war. These standards, or perhaps concepts, are helpful in deciding whether a given use of a weapon would generally be regarded as ethically acceptable. The concepts are sometimes described, in part, as the laws of chivalry. These concepts have certainly existed for very many years and date from a period of limited rather than total warfare: the warfare of armies facing each other on a battlefield. The rules of chivalry include prohibitions of:

1. Treachery.
2. Aggravating the suffering of disabled men.
3. The rendering of death inevitable.
4. The use of poison and poisoned weapons.

These prohibitions all relate to actions and are moral or ethical judgements. However, the list is internally inconsistent in that whilst (1), (2) and (3) define general aspects of behaviour, (4) specifies a particular weapon system or means of killing. These prohibitions form part of the customary rules of war and as such form a part of 'The Rules of War as Recognized by Civilized Nations'. The broad origins of these rules, some detailed aspects of the rules and the implications of their origins will be considered next.

ORIGINS OF THE RULES OF WAR

The generally accepted rules of war, like much other international law, may arise from several sources. These may be divided into:

1. Customary international law which defines how states have behaved over a period of time. Customary law need not make any appeal to ethical thinking; indeed, it may not be rationally based and it is certainly subject to change.
2. Treaty law or conventional law. This is often introduced to reinforce customary law or to create new international law—for example, a boundary change or the agreement between nations to abandon the use of a weapon system.
3. Ethical concepts generally held in common by civilized nations even though they may follow different religions, and, therefore, adhere to different moral codes. Chivalrous behaviour during war is often said to fall into this category.
4. General principles of law as recognized by civilized countries. Some would add the general principles of international law.

Bearing in mind these various sources, five major principles of law as concerns conduct of warfare may be considered.[1]

1. The principle of military necessity. This states that subject to other principles, e.g. of humanity and chivalry, a participant is justified in applying any amount and any kind of force to compel the complete submission of the enemy with the least possible expenditure of life, time and money.
2. The principle of humanity, prohibiting the employment of any kind or degree of violence that is not actually necessary for the purpose of the war.
3. The principle of chivalry, implying concepts of honourable behaviour and mutual respect between forces.
4. The principle of reprisal—or the right to take action which would normally be considered illegal in order to demonstrate that illegal activities on the part of one's opponent will not be tolerated.
5. The principle of self-defence, allowing action to be taken against an actual or impending attack.

Principles 1 and 2 may be considered together: these principles imply much of the accepted rules of how a war should be conducted. They embody the concept that *just wars* are fought to compel one's opponents to amend their actions and not for their annihilation. Under this principle, the disproportionate application of force, destruction of people and property in excess of that needed to achieve the military objective and deliberate extension of the duration of the war are prohibited. No mention is made of individual weapon systems. How CW conforms to these requirements will depend entirely upon how it is used. The use of chemicals *may* represent a use of force disproportionate to the end in view. However, the use of chemical weapons *does not necessarily* represent such a violation of a principle of war; for example, the use of one shell loaded with nerve agent during a tank engagement could not be defined as a use of disproportionate force.

A principle often invoked by those who oppose the use of chemical weapons is that of chivalry, and it is here that we approach the centre of many people's objections to CW. The principles of chivalrous behaviour seem very long-lived and their major prohibitions have already been stated.

Along with the prohibitions listed above, the necessity of providing warning of attacks is generally accepted in theory, but ignored in practice; particularly as regards air raids. To the prohibitions another could be added, embraced in part by the prohibition of the concept of deliberately aggravated suffering—weapons producing suffering but no military advantage should clearly be banned.

Having considered the origins of international law as they affect the conduct of wars, one can consider the commonly made criticisms of CW and ascribe weight to them.

ANALYSIS OF OFTEN-ASSERTED OBJECTIONS TO CHEMICAL WARFARE IN TERMS OF ETHICS AND THE RULES OF WAR

A great many criticisms have been made of CW; some of these will be considered below.

Chemical warfare is uncontrollable

If CW were uncontrollable, then the principle of humanity would clearly be breached. It is important to understand what is meant by uncontrollability of CW. Two possible interpretations exist:

1. The weapons themselves cannot be controlled. This is untrue, as a very great deal is known of the likely spread of chemicals on a battlefield and modern weapons allow more precise targeting than older systems.
2. The second interpretation of uncontrollability is that use would escalate out of control. Given the rules of war, this is no more likely to occur than a loss of control in the use of conventional weapons, e.g. escalation of bombing of civilian populations.

Chemical weapons produce unpredictable effects

This is untrue. Compared with the random chance (real unpredictability) of effects of fragmenting munitions, the effects of chemical weapons may be predicted with considerable accuracy.

Chemical weapons produce inevitable death

This is untrue. During WWI, the mortality in mustard gas casualties was of the order of 2%; over 8% of gunshot wounds resulted in death. High concentrations of lethal agents, such as nerve agents, would likely produce inevitable death, but again this is a criticism of mode of use rather than the weapon.

Chemical weapons produce excessive suffering

Great emphasis was placed during WWI and afterwards on the suffering of gas casualties. The reason for this propaganda drive have already been discussed. The painting by Sargant showing the shuffling line of blinded gas casualties has made a great impression on public opinion. The picture does not reveal that by three weeks later all, or almost all, the casualties would have completely recovered their sight. On the other hand, men blinded by shell splinters do not as a general rule recover their sight. Of course, some chemical weapons have been designed to produce pain and so disable the casualty. Phosgene oxime (one of the 'nettle' gases) works in this way. J. B. S. Haldane made the point that injuries, which often became infected, from shell fragments produced a great deal more pain than the majority of chemical injuries. This is supported by the frequent need for strong analgesics—morphine etc.—in cases of severe physical injury and the observation that such measures are much more rarely required by CW casualties.

Chemical weapons would spread to and devastate civilian populations

During WWI, down-wind drift of gases, particularly chlorine and phosgene (gases released from cylinders), did occur and civilians were affected. The number of civilians affected was comparatively small, but the fact that women and children had been affected was stressed in the anti-CW propaganda. Drifting contamination is a problem in CW and is dependent upon wind and local weather conditions. The objection to CW based on its spread to local civilians is in fact not an objection to CW, but an objection, again, to a particular mode of use or to its use on a particular occasion. CW can be used in such a way—precisely targeted weapons discharging compounds of low volatility producing mainly local contamination—that civilians need not be injured.

The question of civilians being injured during war extends beyond the use of chemical weapons. The concept that *no* civilian casualties should be produced dates from the period of very limited wars involving fairly small armies which chose to fight at some distance from civilian populations. In modern warfare—and particularly in so-called 'total war'—civilians will, inevitably, be injured; indeed, some military actions, e.g. bombing of armaments factories and railway terminals, may always be expected to involve the production of civilian casualties. The ethical position of killing civilians has been considered by Catholic, and other, theologians in terms of the 'double effect' concept.[35] This concept states that if civilians are killed as a result of a justified (just) military engagement, then the deaths of the civilians do not make the act which killed them evil. This argument has been used in the nuclear field,[36] where the killing of civilians as a side-effect of a justifiable attack on a military target has been *not* regarded as evil. It should be said that this argument has struck many as dangerous—as indeed all arguments based on an assertion of 'necessity' strike many as dangerous:

> So spake the Fiend, and with necessity,
> The tyrant's plea, excus'd his devilish deeds.[37]

However, it raises a very interesting ethical question regarding the establishment of an absolute view of the rights and wrongs of a conflict. As said earlier, the concept of the 'just war' is based upon the assertion that one can determine a just cause and then pursue that cause using just means. The just cause is seen as transcending simple gains of territory or influence: one must be, in some way, fighting against evil, and it has to be assumed that one's definition of evil is not only correct but would also be admitted to be correct by one's opponents were they able to take an objective view of their actions. There is nothing within the concept of the *just war* which allows the outcome of the conflict to determine whose was the just cause. This represents a change in thinking from times when a military engagement was seen as an acceptable means of settling a claim, i.e. an assertion of the rightness of one's cause, perhaps to an area of territory. This change in concept has much to do with the charges of unchivalrous behaviour often brought against users and proponents of CW.

Chemical weapons are in some way an unchivalrous means of conducting conflict

The concept of chivalrous behaviour embraces a wide range of attitudes and beliefs regarding how one should behave in conflict. The concept of respect for one's enemy, the belief that one is not *per se* fighting to kill one's enemy but to make his rulers change their ways, and the belief that 'fair play' has some role to play, even in war, all make up a part of the concept of chivalry. The concepts are held to be infringed if one side behaves in a treacherous fashion, i.e. having made an agreement, breaks that agreement. This is a sensible concept, based as it is upon the notion that normal life, i.e. after a war, as well as the rather abnormal life experienced during a war, will be dependent upon one's capacity to trust others. Clearly, a country which has made an agreement not to use chemical weapons and then uses them, e.g. Iraq in the 1980s, could be considered to have acted treacherously. The validity of the allegation is in no part dependent upon the nature of the treacherous act, and the use of chemical weapons cannot *per se* be described as an act of treachery.

The definition of what constitutes a treacherous act is sometimes considerably extended to include acts carried out in a clandestine manner and for which no warning is provided. The idea of a gas seeping along trenches, maiming and killing, conjures up a picture of clandestine activity. There is some dependence here upon the difficulty of detecting an attack by an invisible gas, and this is seen again as a hallmark of a clandestine operation. Surprise is a fundamental concept of military tactics, and warning of an attack upon troops is not required under generally accepted rules of war. Warning of attacks which could involve injury to civilians has been held to be necessary, to allow evacuation of non-combatants, but in the days of rockets and air attacks this requirement is seldom regarded as mandatory.

Concepts of chivalry are also held to be infringed if one acts in a way that does not require some measure of courage, ideally as much courage as shown by one's opponents, and one is therefore not prepared to demonstrate one's willingness to place one's life at risk. Weapons which strike from long range, weapons operated by civilians (in particular scientists) attract censure on these grounds. It is here that we are very close indeed to, or perhaps at, the heart of the widespread objections to CW. When matchlock muskets were introduced it was observed that 'Soldiers were struck down by abominable bullets which had been discharged by cowardly and base knaves, who would never have dared to meet true soldiers face to face.'[20] J. B. S. Haldane noted that Chevalier Bayard (described by contemporaries as 'sans peur et sans raproche') was the soul of courtesy to captured knights, and even bowmen, but invariably put to death musketeers or other users of gunpowder who fell into his hands. During WWI, Lord Kitchener described the German use of CW as an indication of the extent of depravity to which Germany would sink in an attempt to compensate for a lack of courage on the part of her forces.[38] J. B. S. Haldane excoriated such a view, describing it as 'bayardism', and observed that it represented 'one of the most hideous forms of sentimentalism which has ever supported evil upon earth—the attachment of the professional soldier to cruel and obsolete killing machines.'[2]

Chivalrous behaviour also in some way depends upon a balance of forces and capacities to wage war. Two well-matched armies composed of equally well-armed and equally brave troops forms the model for a conflict where chivalrous behaviour is likely to occur. Scientists of one side giving that side an advantage which no amount of courage and bravery on the part of their opponents could counter, particularly if the weapon system providing such an advantage was cheap to produce, is often seen as an example of unchivalrous conduct.

A last point usually included in definitions of chivalrous behaviour is one relating to the use of poisons and poisoned weapons. This is almost invariably seen as wrong—particularly amongst civilized nations. The poisoned weapon is seen as designed to make death inevitable or to produce unnecessary and aggravated suffering and, along with the expanding (dum-dum) bullet and the barbed lance, has long been prohibited. As regards poison, a rational and deep-rooted fear certainly exists in most people. The concepts already mentioned of the lack of need for physical courage on the part of the poisoner and the fact that such an attack may evade detection also add to the particular dislike of this method of killing. In the first section of this account, the intense level of activity of poisoners in the Middle Ages was stressed. The view that poisoning is unchivalrous may stem from the very pragmatic view that unless poisoning were outlawed, no ruler would be safe, and no war could ever be won, for a late 'assault by poison' could reverse any victory acquired on the field of battle. This prohibition, whilst rational and sensible, does not bear upon the large-scale use of chemicals during war, but rather upon the small-scale use of chemicals during peace.

Terrorism

In 1994 and 1995 there were two instances of the use of sarin against civilian populations by terrorists, both in Japan. The first was in Matsumoto, a mountain town in central Japan. Seven people died. There were about 200 casualties who suffered symptoms which were typical of organophosphate poisoning. Treatment was with atropine and diazepam. Oxime reactivators were not used for fear that the poisoning was caused by a carbamate. In March 1995 a similar incident happened on the Tokyo underground subway system. There was a large number of casualties and the incident was similar to the one described above, but the cause of the poisoning was recognized earlier as sarin, and PAM methiodide was used in addition to atropine. There was a total of eight deaths. Myosis, headache and dyspnoea were the most constant signs. The myosis was a very severe and long-lasting one and it was associated with marked discomfort. Cholinesterase levels, which were initially very low, seemed to recover very quickly (within hours), in those successfully resuscitated. Psychological and other sequelae seem to have been few and the hospital staff were rarely affected, despite a lack of individual physical protective clothing.

CONCLUSIONS

The use of chemical weapons is prohibited by a number of international treaties or conventions. This illegality is said to confirm and codify a customary prohibition based on concepts of ethics and morals. Despite these prohibitions, and unlike with other weapons systems which are also prohibited, the number of countries which have acquired or which are acquiring chemical weapons continues to increase. It might be argued that this is explained, in part, by the lack of force of international agreements resulting from their being based upon false assertions and their being established largely as a result of vigorous propaganda exercises in the aftermath of a world war. Current international moves to abandon chemical weapons may well be brought to a successful conclusion but, with the lack of a sound and persuasive argument against the use of such weapons, it remains very unwise to assume that clandestine production of such weapons will not be attempted and that they will not be used during a war. Also, the lack of a sound ethical compulsion to desist from using such weapons may very likely lead to their proliferation and use in the so-called Third World conflicts, particularly amongst nations with no memory of WWI.

REFERENCES

1. General Pershing, US Army (1970) In: *Legal Limits on the Use of Chemical and Biological Weapons* (A Van W Thomas and AJ Thomas, eds). Dallas: Southern Methodist University Press.
2. Haldane JBS (1925) *Callinicus: A Defence of Chemical Warfare*. London: Kegan Paul, French, Trubner & Co. Ltd.
3. Haber F (1919) On the occasion of his being presented with the Nobel Prize for Chemistry. In: *A Higher Form of Killing* (R Harris and J Paxman, eds). London: Chatto and Windus, 1982.
4. Fotion N and Elfstrom G (1986) *Military Ethics*. London: Routledge and Kegan Paul.
5. Robinson JP (1971) The rise of CB weapons. In: *The Problem of Chemical and Biological Warfare*, Chapter 2. New York: Stockholm International Peace Research Institute.
6. The Reprint Society (1938) *The Notebooks of Leonardo da Vinci*. London: The Reprint Society.
7. Blyth AW and Blyth MW (1920) *Poisons: Their Effects and Detection*. London: Charles Griffin & Co. Ltd.
8. Prentiss AM (1937) *Chemicals in War*. New York: McGraw-Hill Book Company Inc.
9. Haber LF (1986) *The Poisonous Cloud—Chemical Warfare in The First World War*. Oxford: Clarendon Press.
10. Holmstedt B (1959) Pharmacology of organophosphorus cholinesterase inhibitors. *Pharmacol Rev*, **11**, 567–688.
11. *Scientific American* (1989) March Issue, p. 8.
12. Mahan AH (1937) In: *Chemicals in War* (AM Prentiss, ed.), p. 686. New York: McGraw-Hill Book Company Inc.
13. US State Department (1937) Statement regarding the First Hague Conference, 1899. In: *Chemicals in War* (AM Prentiss, ed.), p. 685. New York: McGraw-Hill Book Company Inc.
14. Robinson JP (1971) *Popular attitudes towards CBW 1919–1939*. In: *The Problem of Chemical and Biological Warfare*, Chapter 3. New York: Stockholm International Peace Research Institute.
15. French J (1915) Second Battle of Ypres. *The Times*, 12 July, p. 9.
16. *Journal of Industrial and Engineering Chemistry* (1919). Beware the Ide[a]s of March! (Editorial). **11**, 814–816.
17. *The Times* (1921) *A Rain of Death*. 14 March, p. 11.
18. *The Times* (1921) *A Deadly War Gas*. 1 September, p. 9.
19. Lefebure V (1921) *The Riddle of the Rhine*. London: W. Collins Sons & Co. Ltd.
20. Vedder EB (1925) *The Medical Aspects of Chemical Warfare*. Baltimore: Williams and Wilkins Co.
21. Brown FJ (1968) *Chemical Warfare: A Study in Restraints*. Princeton: Greenwood Press.
22. Stockholm International Peace Research Institute (1971) *The Problem of Chemical and Biological Warfare*, Appendix 5. New York: Stockholm International Peace Research Institute.
23. *The Times* (1929) *Civil Population and Gas Warfare*. 20 May, p. 9.
24. *The Times* (1928) *Sham Air Attack on Leningrad: Gas Masks and Bombs*. 11 June, p. 14.
25. Steed W (1934) Aerial warfare: secret German plans. *Nineteenth Century and After*, **116**, 1–15, 331–339.
26. Ministry of Defence (1936) *Air Raid Precautions Handbook No. 1*. London: HMSO.
27. Gilbert M (1991) *Churchill. A Life*, pp. 782–783. London: Heinemann.
28. Meselson M and Robinson JP (1980) Chemical warfare and chemical disarmament. *Sci Am*. **242**, 34–43.

29. Liddell Hart BH (1960) *Deterrent of Defence—A Fresh Look at the West's Military Position*. London: Stevens and Sons, Ltd.
30. McKenna JC (1960) Ethics and war: a Catholic view. *Am Polit Sci Rev*, **54**, 647–658.
31. Haldane JJ (1987) Defence policy, the just war and the intention to deter. *Defence Anal*, **3**, 51–61.
32. Russell B (1927) *An Outline of Western Philosophy*. London: George Allen and Unwin, Ltd.
33. Haldane JJ (1987) *Ethics and Biological Warfare Arms Control*. October Issue, p. 24.
34. Sims NA (1987) *Morality and Biological Warfare Arms Control*. May Issue.
35. Krikus RJ (1964) On the morality of chemical and biological war. *Conflict Resolution*, Vol. IX.
36. Ramsay P (1961) *War and the Christian Conscience*. Durham: Duke University Press.
37. Milton J (1966) *Paradise Lost*. Oxford: Oxford University Press.
38. Letter from General Kitchener to Sir J. French, 1915. (Copy in possession of author.)

2

THE PHYSICOCHEMICAL PROPERTIES AND GENERAL TOXICOLOGY OF CHEMICAL WARFARE AGENTS

Chemical warfare (CW) agents may be encountered as solids, liquids or gases. Some agents, e.g. sulphur mustard, may appear as solids under North European winter conditions (freezing point 14.4°C), as a liquid at a wide range of temperatures (boiling point 219°C) or as a vapour evaporating from the liquid phase.

CW agents may also be encountered as mixtures or solutions of one agent in another, or of an agent in a solvent. The mixing of lewisite with sulphur mustard has been undertaken to lower the vapour pressure and freezing point of the mustard and hence to increase its persistence, without reducing the effective CW payload of weapon systems. Sulphur mustard has also been mixed with phenyldichlorarsine, the mixture being referred to as Winterlost, i.e. winter mustard.

BEHAVIOUR OF LIQUID AGENTS

Classical CW agents are, in the main, volatile liquids at ordinary temperatures (phosgene is an exception: a gas at ordinary temperatures). The degree of volatility varies, of course, from compound to compound. The relationship between the liquid and the vapour phase is particularly important in explaining the effect of temperature on the damage likely to be produced by exposure to an agent and to calculations of the persistency of agents. The relationship between the liquid phase and gas (or vapour) phase of a volatile substance is defined by the vapour pressure of that substance.

If a sample of a volatile liquid is placed in an enclosed space, evaporation will take place: molecules leave the liquid phase and enter the gas phase at the surface of the liquid. Molecules also leave the gas phase and re-enter the liquid phase.

Equilibrium is reached when molecules leave and re-enter the liquid phase at the same rate. In the equilibrium state the air above the liquid is said to be saturated with vapour, and that vapour to exert the saturated vapour pressure (SVP) characteristic of the liquid at the given temperature.

The SVP of a liquid defines its volatility: the higher the SVP, the greater the volatility of the compound. When the SVP is equal to the atmospheric pressure, the liquid boils. The SVP of water at $100°C = 760$ mmHg. It is common knowledge that water boils at a lower temperature at high altitude than at sea level. This is because the SVP becomes equal to the reduced atmospheric pressure at high altitude at a temperature of less than $100°C$. Of course, air is not always saturated with water vapour. When saturation is complete, the pressure exerted by the vapour is the SVP. The relative humidity (RH) of air defines the extent of saturation. Air at an RH of 80% contains sufficient water vapour to exert a pressure equal to 80% of the SVP at the specified temperature.

$$\text{RH} = \frac{\text{Actual vapour pressure}}{\text{SVP}} \times 100\%$$

The SVP of a substance is dependent upon temperature: the greater the temperature, the greater the SVP. The SVP of a substance at a particular temperature may be determined by use of Regnault's equation:

$$\log_{10} p = A + B/(273 + t)$$

where A and B are constants which vary from compound to compound and t is the temperature in degrees Celsius. Values of A and B may be calculated from determinations of the boiling points of the substance, t_1 and t_2, at two different pressures, p_1 and p_2. A pair of simultaneous equations is produced:

$$\log_{10} p_1 = A + B/(273 + t_1)$$
$$\log_{10} p_2 = A + B/(273 + t_2)$$

The equations may be solved for A and B. The equation describing the relationship between SVP and temperature for sulphur mustard is:

$$\log_{10} p = 8.3937 - 2734.5/(273 + t)$$

Standard values for the constants A and B for a number of CW agents are given in Table 1.

The SVP of a compound is dependent only upon temperature; it is important to remember that it is independent of barometric pressure. Of course, the gas and liquid phases of a substance must be in contact for these rules to apply.

If a quantity of water is introduced into an evacuated container at $37°C$, evaporation will occur and the pressure in the container will rise to 47 mmHg: the SVP of water is $37°C$.

If a quantity of water is introduced into a closed container of dry air at $37°C$ and atmospheric pressure (760 mmHg), the water will evaporate until the pressure exerted by the water vapour in the container equals the SVP of water at $37°C$, i.e. 47 mmHg. The pressure in the container will be $760 + 47 = 807$ mmHg.

Table 1. Constants for calculating vapour pressure
using shorter form of Regnault's equation

Compound	A	B
Phosgene	7.5595	−1326
Chloropicrin	8.2424	−2045.1
Cyanogen bromide	10.3282	−2457.5
Dichlordiethylene sulphide	8.3937	−2734.5
Methyl dichlorarsine	8.6944	−2281.7
Diphenyl chloroarsine	7.8930	−3288

(After Sartori 1939)

If, on the other hand, the contents of the container were maintained at atmospheric pressure, by allowing the container to expand, then the water vapour would still come to exert a pressure of 47 mmHg, the other gases exerting a pressure of 713 mmHg (changes assumed to take place isothermally). The gases other than water vapour would obey Dalton's law of partial pressures and would each exert a partial pressure in accordance with the volume proportion occupied by the gas in question, e.g.

Partial pressure of oxygen $PO_2 = 0.2093 \times 713 = 149.2$ mmHg

This is an important fact in respiratory physiology: the PO_2 of dry air is 159.1 mmHg but the PO_2 of moist air in the trachea is 149.2 mmHg.

The concentration of a substance in the vapour phase (saturated vapour concentration: SVC) may be calculated from the SVP of the substance. This may be done to a useful level of accuracy by the simple application of the ideal gas law. Table 2 specifies the symbols and units of the parameters used in the calculation.

Consider sulphur mustard at 40°C:

$$SVP = 0.45 \text{ mmHg}$$
$$= 0.45 \times 101\,325/760 \text{ N m}^{-2}$$

Table 2. Terms, symbols and units needed for the calculation
of SVC from the ideal gas law

Symbol	Term	Units
P	Pressure	$N\ m^{-2}$
V	Volume	m^3
n	Number of moles of gas present per m^3	
T	Absolute temperature	K
R	Gas constant: 8.3143	$N\ m\ K^{-1}\ mol^{-1}$

By the ideal gas law:

$$PV = nRT$$

$$n = \frac{PV}{RT}$$

$$n = 0.45 \times \frac{101\,325}{760} \times \frac{1}{8.3143} \times \frac{1}{313} \text{ mol m}^{-3}$$

Gram molecular weight of sulphur mustard $= 159$ g
1 mol $= 159$ g

$$\therefore \text{SVC} = \frac{0.45 \times 101\,325 \times 159}{760 \times 8.3143 \times 313} = 3.67 \text{ g m}^{-3}$$

i.e. in the units most commonly used in thinking about CW agents, at 40°C the maximum concentration of sulphur mustard (the saturated vapour concentration) $=$ 3670 mg m^{-3}.

This result can also be obtained by arguing as follows:

1 mole of any gas at STP occupies 22.4 litres
At 40°C, assuming barometric pressure $= 760$ mmHg,
1 mole of sulphur mustard would occupy $(273 + 40)/273 = 25.68$ litres

It is important to understand what the last statement means: 159 g of sulphur mustard vapour constrained to occupy 25.68 litres would exert a pressure of 760 mmHg. However, we know that the SVP of sulphur mustard at 40°C $=$ 0.45 mmHg, i.e. the 159 g of sulphur mustard exert a pressure of 0.45 mmHg rather than 760 mmHg. The volume occupied by the 159 g of sulphur mustard vapour must then be:

$$25.68 \times 760/0.45 = 43\,370 \text{ litres}$$

i.e. 43 370 litres of air saturated with sulphur mustard at 40°C contain 159 g of sulphur mustard,

or: 1 litre of air saturated with sulphur mustard at 40°C contains 159/43 370 $=$ 0.00367 g of sulphur mustard,

or: 1 m^3 of air saturated with sulphur mustard at 40°C contains 3.67 g or 3670 mg of sulphur mustard,

i.e. the SVC of sulphur mustard is 3670 mg m^{-3}.

Use is also made of SVP in calculating the persistency (or persistence) of CW agents. Classically, the persistence of a CW agent has been compared to that of water at 15°C, and its value, S, indicates that the compound would take S times as long as water to evaporate at 15°C.

Table 3. Persistences of some war gases

	Temperature (°C)								
	−10	−5	0	+5	+10	+15	+20	+25	+30
Phosgene	0.014	0.012	0.01	0.008	—	—	—	—	—
Chloropicrin	1.36	0.98	0.72	0.54	0.4	0.3	0.23	0.18	0.14
Trichloromethyl chloroformate	2.7	1.9	1.4	1.0	0.7	0.5	0.4	0.3	0.2
Lewisite	96	63.1	42.1	28.5	19.6	13.6	9.6	6.9	5
Dichloroethyl sulphide (liquid)	—	—	—	—	—	103	67	44	29
Dichloroethyl sulphide (solid)	2400	1210	630	333	181	—	—	—	—
Bromobenzyl cyanide	6930	4110	2490	1530	960	610	395	260	173

From Sartori.

S is given by:

$$S = \frac{p_1}{p} \sqrt{\frac{M_1 T}{M T_1}}$$

where:

S = persistence

p_1 = vapour pressure of water at 15°C (288 K) = 12.7 mmHg

p = vapour pressure of substance in question at T K

M_1 = molecular weight of water = 18

M = molecular weight of substance in question

T = Absolute temperature

T_1 = Absolute temperature corresponding to 15°C, i.e. 288 K

Table 3 shows the persistence of some CW agents.

Differences between values quoted by different authorities for the SVP of sulphur mustard have led to a range of values being quoted for its persistence. The value given in Table 3 is of more use as a comparison with those of the other agents listed than as an absolute value.

BEHAVIOUR OF SOLUTIONS OF AGENTS

The above discussion has been concerned, in the main, with the vapour pressures produced by pure liquids. However, two other conditions should be considered:

1. Solutions of a volatile liquid in a solvent.
2. Solutions of a gas or gases in a solvent.

Solutions of a volatile liquid in a solvent

If a volatile liquid A is dissolved in a solvent it will continue to exert a vapour pressure, though this will be less than that which would be exerted at the same temperature by a pure sample of A. The change in vapour pressure, for ideal solutions (i.e. a solution in which the cohesive forces are identical to those which would obtain in the pure samples of the separate components of the solution), is defined by Raoult's Law:

> The partial vapour pressure of A in a solution, at a given temperature, is equal to the vapour pressure of pure A, at the same temperature, multiplied by the mole fraction of A in the solution.

If both solute A and solvent B are volatile, then the total vapour pressure will be the sum of that exerted by A and by B.

In practice, many solutions of liquids in liquids do not act as ideal solutions and the total vapour pressure above the solution may be greater than or less than that predicted by Raoult's law.

Solution of a gas or gases in a solvent

The amount of a gas which will dissolve in a volume of solvent is dependent upon a number of factors:

- The partial pressure of the gas to which the solvent is exposed. Henry's Law states: 'The mass of gas dissolved by a given volume of liquid at a constant temperature is proportional to the pressure of the gas.'
- The solubility of the gas in the liquid: the Bunsen coefficient defines the volume of gas which dissolves, at STP, in unit volume of solvent at one atmosphere gas pressure.
- The temperature at which the solution is formed. The solubility of most gases decreases as temperature rises.

Gases dissolved in liquids are often described as exerting a partial pressure 'in the liquid'; for example, the partial pressure of oxygen in arterial blood is 100 mmHg. This means that the amount of oxygen in physical solution in a unit volume of blood is equal to that which would be dissolved in a unit volume of blood equilibrated with oxygen at a pressure of 100 mmHg, or with air containing oxygen exerting a partial pressure of 100 mmHg.

It is important to remember that though the *partial pressure* of a gas in a liquid may be low, the *content* of gas in the solution may be high. Comroe[1] has pointed out that 'It is possible ... to have more millilitres of a very soluble gas in 1 litre of liquid than in 1 litre of a gas mixture on top of it at equilibrium (equal partial pressures).'

BEHAVIOUR OF AEROSOLS

As well as appearing as liquid, e.g. splashes or large droplets, CW agents may be encountered as aerosols. An aerosol has been defined by Muir:[2]

> The word aerosol is a general name referring to any atmosphere containing particles which remain airborne for a reasonable length of time and is used to describe all particles that can be inhaled whether they are therapeutic, industrial, or of natural origin such as bacteria, fungi and pollens.

A more formal definition is:

> An aerosol is a colloid system in which the continuous phase (dispersion medium) is a gas.

Green and Lane[3] have pointed out that the term 'aerosol' was coined by Professor F. G. Donnan towards the end of World War I. The term was intended to describe the sort of system exemplified by the irritant arsenical smokes then being developed. It should be recalled that though the term aerosol was intended as a counterpart to the term hydrosol, used to describe liquid colloid suspensions, the analogy has always been imperfect in that an aerosol is inherently unstable in comparison with a hydrosol. Green and Lane included dusts of small particle size, smokes and some mists within their use of the term aerosol: their criterion being that the particle size should be sufficiently small to 'confer some degree of stability, at any rate as far as sedimentation is concerned'.[3]

A common example of an aerosol is provided by fog. If the temperature of a mass of air containing water vapour falls below the temperature of saturation, condensation of water onto the surface of dust particles will occur, and fog will be formed. Table 4 shows the water content of air saturated with water at different temperatures.

Table 4. SVP and water content of air at various temperatures

Temp. (°C)	Vapour pressure (mmHg)	Water content $(g\ m^{-3})$
0	4.57	4.87
10	9.14	9.36
20	17.36	17.15
30	31.51	30.08
40	54.87	50.67

If air saturated with water vapour at 30°C is cooled to 10°C, then some 20 g of water will be condensed from each cubic metre of air. Under suitable conditions the water forms fog. If only the layer of air adjacent to the ground cools, e.g. during the night, dew forms. The dew point is defined as the temperature of saturation of the air with water vapour. For example, air 60% saturated with water at 40°C will contain approximately 33 g of water per m³. Such content is equivalent to 100% saturation at 32°C. If the air is cooled, water will begin to condense as the temperature falls below 32°C, i.e. the dewpoint of the air is 32°C.

FATE OF LIQUID AEROSOLS

It may be shown that the vapour pressure exerted by a convex surface is greater than that exerted by a plane surface.[4] This effect of the curvature of the surface is referred to as the Kelvin effect, and is of importance in considering the stability of small liquid droplets. If a very small droplet occurs in an atmosphere in which the vapour pressure is the maximum associated with a plane surface (SVP), evaporation from the surface of the droplet will still occur as a result of the vapour pressure exerted by the droplet surface exceeding SVP. As the droplet becomes smaller, so the curvature of the surface increases and evaporation continues. This effect in part explains the observation that a dust-free vapour does not form droplets at a temperature below the normal temperature of condensation (the dew point). The Kelvin effect must be taken into account when considering the stability of small liquid aerosol droplets in the airways.

Table 5 shows the time taken (in seconds) for water droplets of different sizes to evaporate completely.[5]

If, on the other hand, a droplet of a watery solution which exerts a SVP less than that of pure water is exposed to air saturated with water vapour, it will grow in size. Such growth is described as hygroscopic growth. Hygroscopic growth is a complex topic but may be usefully approached in a series of stages.

Table 5. Survival time of water droplets of varying size in air at varying relative humidity

Droplet diameter (μm)	Per cent relative humidity			
	0	25	50	75
1	0.29×10^{-4}	0.39×10^{-4}	0.58×10^{-4}	1.18×10^{-4}
2	1.16×10^{-4}	1.55×10^{-4}	2.3×10^{-4}	4.7×10^{-4}
5	7.3×10^{-4}	9.7×10^{-4}	1.5×10^{-3}	2.9×10^{-3}
10	2.9×10^{-3}	3.9×10^{-4}	5.8×10^{-3}	1.2×10^{-2}
20	1.16×10^{-2}	1.6×10^{-2}	2.4×10^{-2}	4.7×10^{-2}
90	0.25	0.3	0.5	1.0

Time in seconds.
From Florey (1962).

All solutions considered in the section are assumed to be watery and dilute.

Consider a small droplet of water exposed to an excess of dry air. Evaporation from the surface of the droplet will occur. As the droplet becomes very small, the rate of evaporation will increase as a result of the Kelvin effect.

Consider a small droplet of water exposed to air saturated with water vapour. Evaporation from the surface of the droplet will occur as a result of the Kelvin effect.

Consider a droplet of solution of a non-volatile solute exerting a vapour pressure of less than the air to which it is exposed. The droplet will grow as a result of water condensing onto its surface. The concentration of the solution comprising the droplet will fall and the vapour pressure exerted by that solution will rise. Once the vapour pressure exerted by the solution equals the vapour pressure of the air, the droplet is described as stable. One might wonder, given what has been said regarding the Kelvin effect, how a droplet could ever be described as stable. The Kelvin effect is, however, decreasingly important as the droplet grows, and exerts so small an effect on droplets of >15 μm diameter that these droplets are, in practice, stable.

Given that the droplet is of a stable size, i.e. in equilibrium at a given relative humidity, the concentration of a given solute in the droplet may be calculated. Cocks and Fernando calculated that droplets containing a 20% solution of sulphuric acid would be in equilibrium at a relative humidity of 88% and a temperature of 37°C.[6]

The equilibrium size of a droplet may be related to its original size by means of an equation derived by Ferron:

$$\frac{d_e}{d_0} = \left(\frac{\rho_0}{\rho_e}[1 + M_w iH/M_0(K - H)]\right)^{1/3}$$

where:

d_e = equilibrium diameter

d_0 = initial diameter

ρ_0 = initial density of droplet

ρ_e = equilibrium density of droplet

M_w = molecular weight of solute

M_0 = molecular weight of water

H = relative humidity

i = number of ions produced on dissociation of a molecule of solute

K = constant determined by the Kelvin equation :

$$K = \exp\left(\frac{4\sigma M_w}{RT\rho_e d_e}\right)$$

where in addition:

σ = surface tension

R = the gas constant

T = absolute temperature

Evaporation is accompanied by local cooling and condensation by local warming. The addition of mass to droplets and the conduction of latent heat away from the surface of the droplet or particle are, as has been pointed out by Pritchard, the determining processes of particle growth.[7] Under conditions of turbulent airflow, conduction of heat away from the surface of droplets or particles is enhanced and hygroscopic growth rates exceed those found under still conditions or under conditions of laminar airflow. The implications of this will be considered later.

The importance of droplet growth under the close to saturated conditions obtaining in the respiratory tract is considerable. The pattern of deposition of particles or droplets in the respiratory tract is dependent upon particle or droplet size, and growth of particles or droplets will affect the pattern of deposition. This will also be considered further below.

MATHEMATICAL DESCRIPTION OF AEROSOLS

(In this section the term 'particles' should be taken to mean both solid particles and liquid droplets.)

Though aerosols containing particles of uniform size (monodisperse aerosols) can be prepared experimentally, naturally occurring aerosols contain particles of varying size. Such aerosols are described as polydisperse. If the particles found in such an aerosol are sampled and measured, then the distribution of particle size may be determined. Studies by Green[8] demonstrated that the distribution of particle size tended to be skewed, there being many more small than large particles. Drinker[9] showed that the typical skewed distribution curve could be transformed into a normal or Gaussian distribution curve by plotting the logarithm of the particle diameter against the percentage of the total aerosol made up by particles of different sizes. This represented a great step forward in thinking about particle size in aerosol clouds: its importance cannot be overestimated. To understand the terms used to describe particle size, a revision of the theory of normal and log-normal distribution curves may be helpful.

The normal distribution curve is described by the equation:

$$n = \frac{\sum n}{\sigma\sqrt{2\pi}}\, e^{[-(x-m)^2/2\sigma^2]}$$

where n is the frequency of observations of the value x, $\sum n$ is the total number of observations, m is the arithmetic mean and σ is the standard deviation.

The arithmetic mean is given by:

$$m = \frac{\sum(nx)}{\sum n}$$

and the standard deviation by:

$$\sigma = \sqrt{\frac{\sum[n(x-m)^2]}{\sum n}}$$

Similarly, in the log-normal distribution the mean (now the logarithmic or geometric mean) m_g is given by:

$$\log m_g = \frac{\sum (n \log x)}{\sum n}$$

and the logarithmic or geometric standard deviation by:

$$\log \sigma_g = \sqrt{\frac{\sum [n(\log x - \log m_g)^2]}{\sum n}}$$

In the case of a normal distribution the arithmetic mean, the median and the mode are identical. Similarly, in a log-normal distribution the geometric mean, the geometric median and the geometric mode are identical. Of course, in a log-normal distribution the arithmetic mean, the arithmetic median and the arithmetic mode all differ one from another. This is shown in Figures 1 and 2.

The geometric mean (m_g) of a log-normal distribution may be shown to be identical with the arithmetic median of that distribution. The arithmetic mean and arithmetic mode of a log-normal distribution are related to the geometric mean. The following equations define the relationships:

$$\log \text{median} = \log m_g$$
$$\log \text{mean} = \log m_g + 1.1513 \, \log^2 \sigma_g$$
$$\log \text{mode} = \log m_g - 2.3026 \, \log^2 \sigma_g$$

The constants preceding the $\log^2 \sigma_g$ terms are the result of conversion from natural logarithms to logarithms of base 10 ($\ln x = 2.3026 \log x$).

It should be understood that log mean is the log of the arithmetic mean and not the logarithmic mean. To avoid confusion we shall use the term geometric mean in place of logarithmic mean.

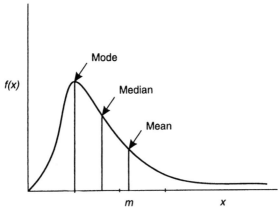

Figure 1. Log-normal distribution showing relationship between mode, mean and median

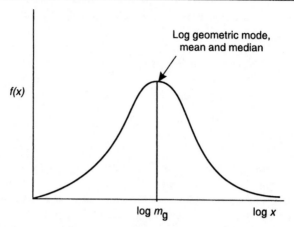

Figure 2. Log-normal distribution plotted with a log scale on the x-axis. Note that the distribution is now normalized, with the geometric mean, median and mode coinciding

Let the geometric mean (m_g) of the distribution of particle sizes in an aerosol be 1.0 μm. Let the geometric standard deviation (σ_g) be 2.0 μm. The arithmetic median (usually referred to simply as the median) of the distribution is then 1.0 μm.

The arithmetic mean (usually referred to as the mean) is given by:

$$\log \text{mean} = \log m_g + 1.1513 \log^2 \sigma_g$$
$$\log \text{mean} = 0 + (1.1513 \times 0.3010 \times 0.3010)$$
$$\log \text{mean} = 0.1043$$
$$\text{mean} = a \ \log 0.1043$$
$$\text{mean} = 1.27 \ \mu\text{m}$$

[Note that $\log^2 \sigma_g = (\log \sigma_g)^2$ and not $\log \sigma_g^2$]

Similarly the arithmetic mode (usually referred to as the mode) is given by:

$$\log \text{mode} = \log m_g - 2.3026 \log^2 \sigma_g$$
$$\log \text{mode} = 0 - (2.3026 \times 0.3010 \times 0.3010)$$
$$\log \text{mode} = -0.2086$$
$$\text{mode} = 0.619 \ \mu\text{m}$$

These values are shown in Figure 3 from Raabe.[10]

The scale on the y-axis of Figure 3 has been devised to standardize this sort of plot. The individual values on the scale on the y-axis are dependent upon the range of particle sizes in the aerosol. If all the particles are between 0 and 1.0 μm in diameter, then the figures on the y-axis may exceed 1.0. If, on the other hand, there is a wide range of particle sizes, the figures on the scale on the y-axis will be very much less than 1.0. Hinds (personal communication) has commented that the values on the

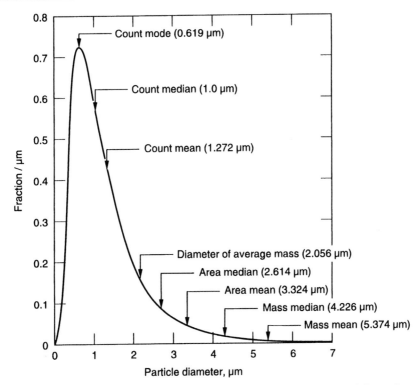

Figure 3. An example of the log-normal distribution function in normalized linear form for CMD = 1.0 and σ_g = 2.0, showing the mode, median and mean of the size distribution, the surface area distribution median and mean diameters, the mass distribution median and mean diameters, and the diameter of average mass. Reproduced with permission from Raabe OG (1970) Generation and characterisation of aerosols. In *Inhalation Carcinogenesis* (MG Hanna, P Nettersheim and JR Gilbert, eds), pp. 123–172. Proceedings of a Biology Division, Oak Ridge National Laboratory Conference. Oak Ridge Tennessee: US Atomic Energy Commission

faction per micrometre scale do not convey any immediate intensive or physical meaning. In Hinds' account,[11] a distribution is shown in which particle size ranges from 0 to 50 μm. The values on the fraction per micrometre scale range from 0 to 0.1. In Figure 3, the distribution of particle size is less broad, 0–6 μm, and the values on the scale on the y-axis range from 0 to 0.8.

The second great advance in the understanding of the distribution of particle sizes in aerosol clouds was reported by Hatch and Choate in 1929.[12] These workers showed that if the logarithm of particle diameter was plotted against the fractional percentage of total mass contributed by particles of different sizes, then a log-normal distribution of identical geometric standard deviation to that of the distribution obtained by plotting the logarithm of particle diameter against percentage frequency was obtained. Raabe[10] summarized this:

any characteristic of the particles in a population which is proportional to the qth power of the diameter can also be described by a log-normal distribution of the same geometric standard deviation as the size distribution and with a median diameter given by:

$$\ln D_q = \ln \text{CMD} + q(\ln \sigma_g)^2$$

Here CMD stands for count median diameter, i.e. m_g in the equations given above.

Mass is proportional to volume and hence to the third power of diameter of a spherical particle. Hence we see:

$$\ln \text{MMD} = \ln \text{CMD} + 3 \ln^2 \sigma_g$$

or to the base 10:

$$\log \text{MMD} = \log \text{CMD} + 6.9078 \log^2 \sigma_g$$

where MMD = mass median diameter.

Similarly, considering surface area:

$$\ln \text{AMD} = \ln \text{CMD} + 2 \ln^2 \sigma_g$$
$$\log \text{AMD} = \log \text{CMD} + 4.6052 \log^2 \sigma_g$$

MMD and area median diameter (AMD) are the geometric means of the mass and area distributions respectively. In the same way that the arithmetic mean and mode were calculated from m_g (count median diameter), so equivalent values can be calculated from MMD and AMD.

In the example given above (CMD (m_g) = 1.0 μm; σ_g = 2.0 μm):

$$\log \text{MMD} = \log m_g + 6.9078 \log^2 \sigma_g$$
$$\log \text{MMD} = 0 + 0.6259$$
$$\text{MMD} = 4.226 \ \mu\text{m}$$
$$\log \text{AMD} = \log m_g + 4.6052 \ \log^2 \sigma_g$$
$$\text{AMD} = 2.614 \ \mu\text{m}$$
$$\log \text{mass mean diameter} = \log \text{MMD} + 1.1513 \ \log^2 \sigma_g$$
$$\text{mass mean diameter} = 5.374 \ \mu\text{m}$$
$$\log \text{mass mode diameter} = \log \text{MMD} - 2.3026 \ \log^2 \sigma_g$$
$$\text{mass mode diameter} = 2.6136 \ \mu\text{m}$$
$$\log \text{area mean diameter} = \log \text{AMD} + 1.1513 \ \log^2 \sigma_g$$
$$\text{area mean diameter} = 3.324 \ \mu\text{m}$$
$$\log \text{area mode diameter} = \log \text{AMD} = 2.3026 \ \log^2 \sigma_g$$
$$\text{area mode diameter} = 1.617 \ \mu\text{m}$$

The mass mode (or modal) diameter and the area mode (or modal) diameter are not much used in describing aerosols; the other calculated parameters are shown in Figure 3.

In addition to the parameters discussed above, Hatch and Choate[12] gave equations which allowed the calculation of the parameters of 'average particle size' introduced by Green.[8] These parameters sound confusingly similar to, but are in fact quite different from, those described above. The following discussion is based on Hinds' outstandingly clear account.[11]

Consider 100 spheres, say apples, of different sizes.

Weigh the 100 apples and divide by 100.

The value obtained is the average mass.

Taking the density of apple as 1, the diameter of a hypothetical apple of average mass could be calculated.

The value obtained is the 'diameter of average mass'.

This approach is described as unweighted: no account has been taken of the distribution of masses and a very misleading result would be obtained if the 100 spheres were not in fact apples but 99 grapes and one pumpkin. However, the method entailed no more than counting the number of spheres and weighing all the spheres together.

Consider, alternatively, measuring the diameters of all the spheres.

Divide the sum of the diameters by 100.

The value obtained is the arithmetic mean diameter. An approximation could be reached by allocating the spheres into categories defined by size, and counting the number in each category counted. Using standard statistical terminology the arithmetic mean diameter would be given by:

$$\bar{d} = \frac{\sum n_i d_i}{N}$$

In this process, the characteristic diameter for each group is weighted by n_i/N, or the fraction of the total number in that size group.

The same approach could be taken for mass and the characteristic diameters of each group weighted by m_i/M, the fraction of the total mass in the size group. Let the average diameter calculated in this way be the mass mean diameter d_{mm}; this will be given by:

$$d_{mm} = \frac{\sum m_i d_i}{M}$$

The mass mean diameter will not equal the diameter of average mass. Hinds' definition[11] is useful:

In the calculation of the diameter of average mass, a coarse and fine particle are given equal representation in the averaging process but the quantity averaged is the mass. In calculating the mass mean diameter, the quantity averaged is the diameter, but it is weighted according to its mass contribution.

Similarly, diameter of average surface should not be confused with surface mean diameter.

Equations for calculating 'average diameters' are given in Table 6, taken from Hatch.[13]

The diameter of average mass (D) of the distribution discussed above may be calculated as follows:

$$\log D = \log m_g + 3.4539 \ \log^2 \sigma_g$$
$$D = 2.056 \ \mu m$$

This parameter is shown in Figure 3. The reader may think it fortunate that diameters of average mass and surface are little used in inhalation toxicology.

If the log-normal distribution of particle size is plotted so that the cumulative frequency appears on the y-axis and the log of the particle diameter on the x-axis, an ogive is produced (Figure 4). This curve may be converted to a straight line by manipulating the scale on the y-axis. If this scale is distributed according to the normal distribution curve, then a straight line will be obtained when the data shown in Figure 4 are plotted (Figure 5). Such a plot is described as a 'log-probability plot' and will be discussed in more detail when the use of probit analysis is considered.

It is worth considering how the geometric standard deviation of the distribution may be derived from this sort of plot. This may be approached by recalling the normal distribution curve obtained when a log-normal distribution is plotted as shown in Figure 6. It will be recalled that in a normal distribution 68% of the observations lie between $+1$ and -1 standard deviations of the mean. In Figure 6 it is shown that 68% of the observations fall between $\log x_a$ and $\log x_b$.

$\log x_b - \log m_g$ (or, equally, $\log m_g - \log x_a$) is the standard deviation of this distribution of $\log x$

antilog ($\log x_b - \log m_g$) is the geometric standard deviation of the distribution of x

antilog ($\log x_b - \log m_g$) = x_b/m_g
antilog ($\log m_g - \log x_a$) = m_g/x_a

thus the geometric standard deviation σ_g is given by:

$$\sigma_g = \frac{x_b}{m_g} = \frac{m_g}{x_a}$$

Figures 4 and 5 show how σ_g may be derived from cumulative frequency plots of the distribution of $\log x$.

From Figure 5 it will be seen that:

$$\sigma_g = \text{antilog} \ (\log x_b - \log m_g) = x_b/m_g = 84\% \ \text{size/50\% size}$$

σ_g is often defined in this way.

Table 6. Mathematical definitions of the average diameters of non-uniform particulate substances in terms of the parameters of the distribution curves by count and by weight

Average diameter	Symbol	Mathematical definition	Equivalent logarithmic value in terms of statistical parameters of distribution curves	
			By count (M_g and σ_g)	By weight (screen analysis) (M_g' and σ_g')
Geometric mean	M_g	$\text{antilog}\left(\dfrac{\sum n \log d}{\sum n}\right)$	$\log M_g$	$\log M_g' - 6.9078 \log^2 \sigma_g'$
Arithmetic mean	δ	$\dfrac{\sum nd}{\sum n}$	$\log M_g + 1.1513 \log^2 \sigma_g$	$\log M_g' - 5.7565 \log^2 \sigma_g'$
Specific surface	d_s	$\left(\dfrac{\sum nd^{-1}}{\sum n}\right)^{-1}$	$\log M_g - 1.1513 \log^2 \sigma_g$	$\log M_g' - 8.0591 \log^2 \sigma_g'$
Surface area	Δ	$\left(\dfrac{\sum nd^2}{\sum n}\right)^{1/2}$	$\log M_g + 2.3026 \log^2 \sigma_g$	$\log M_g' - 4.6052 \log^2 \sigma_g'$
Volume	D	$\left(\dfrac{\sum nd^3}{\sum n}\right)^{1/3}$	$\log M_g + 3.4539 \log^2 \sigma_g$	$\log M_g' - 3.4539 \log^2 \sigma_g'$
Surface* area per unit volume	D^3/Δ^2	$\dfrac{\sum nd^3}{\sum nd^2}$	$\log M_g + 5.7565 \log^2 \sigma_g$	$\log M_g' - 1.1513 \log^2 \sigma_g'$

* This diameter gives the specific surface for the sample as a whole; it should not be confused with d_s, the diameter of the hypothetical particle having *average* specific surface.
From Hatch 1933.

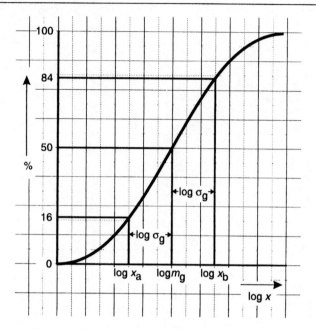

Figure 4. Cumulative plot of a log-normal distribution

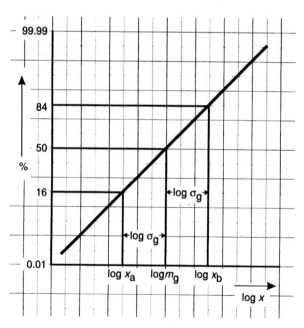

Figure 5. Log-normal distribution plotted on 'log-probability' paper

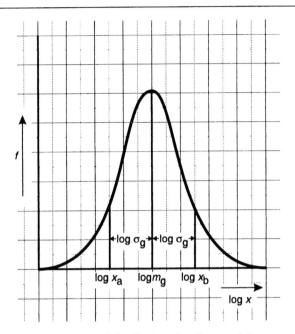

Figure 6. Log-normal distribution plotted on semi-log paper

σ_g may also be calculated as follows:

$$\sigma_g = \frac{xb}{m_g} = \frac{m_g}{xa}$$

$$\sigma_g^2 = \frac{xb}{m_g} x \frac{m_g}{xa} = \frac{xb}{xa}$$

$$\sigma_g = \sqrt{\frac{xb}{xa}}$$

The geometric standard deviation controls the width of the distribution curve plotted as in Figure 6 and the slope of the distribution curve plotted as in Figure 5.

To simplify plotting of data as shown in Figure 5, special log-probability graph paper is used. As an example, the data shown in Table 7 have been plotted on this type of graph paper in Figure 7. σ_g has been calculated from:

$$\sigma_g = \sqrt{\frac{84\% \text{ size}}{16\% \text{ size}}} = 2.08$$

$$m_g = 4.45 \ \mu m$$

Table 7. Distribution of particle size in a sample of particles

Group size (filar units)*	Upper limit of group† (μm)	Group frequency f	Number < upper limit of group size	% < upper limit of group size
1–2	2.3	28	28	18
2–3	3.3	32	60	39
3–4	4.4	20	80	52
4–5	5.5	15	95	62
5–6	6.6	14	109	71
6–7	7.7	8	117	76
7–8	8.8	9	126	82
8–9	9.9	5	131	85
9–10	11.0	4	135	88
10–11	12.1	5	140	91
11–12	13.2	3	143	93
12–13	14.3	2	145	94
13–14	15.4	1	146	95
14–15	16.5	0	146	95
15–16	17.6	2	148	96
16–17	18.7	0	148	96
17–18	19.8	1	149	97
18–19	20.9	0	149	97
19–20	22.0	2	151	98
20–21	23.1	0	151	98
21–22	24.2	0	151	98
22–23	25.3	1	152	99
23–24	26.4	2	154	100

* By calibration, one filar unit = 1.1 μm.
† Note the upper limit of group size is used in plotting cumulative frequency distribution curves. The group midpoints are used in plotting histograms and non-cumulative distribution curves.
After Drinker P and Hatch T (1954) *Industrial Dust*, 2nd edn. McGraw-Hill.

It has already been stated that σ_g is identical for plots of the distribution of any parameter related to particle diameter, e.g. mass or surface area. Log-probability plots of count distribution, surface area distribution and mass distribution against particle diameter would, therefore, be expected to generate parallel lines. This is the case, as shown in Figure 8 (modified from Menzel and Amdur[14]).

The data upon which these curves are based were obtained by use of a cascade impactor, which sizes particles according to their aerodynamic characteristics. The aerodynamic diameter of a particle is the diameter of a spherical particle of unit density which, when falling, reaches the same terminal velocity as the particle in question. This will be discussed further below.

From Figure 8 it will be seen that only 10% of the particles in the aerosol were greater than 1 μm in diameter but that these accounted for about 80% of the total mass of the particles in the aerosol. More dramatically, 50% of the mass was made

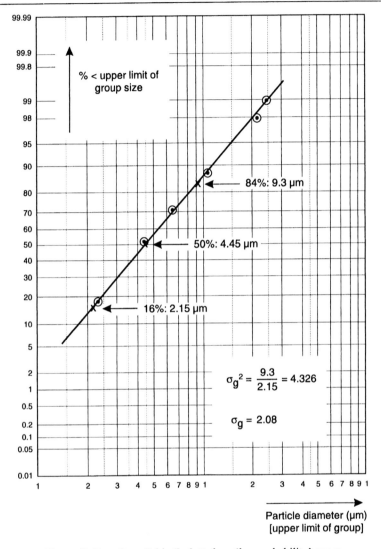

Figure 7. Data from Table 7 plotted on 'log-probability' paper

up by particles of diameter greater than 1.39 μm (mass median diameter $= 1.39$ μm) but these comprised only about 4% of the particles in the aerosol.

DEPOSITION OF AIRBORNE PARTICLES IN THE RESPIRATORY TRACT

A proportion of all inhaled particles deposit in the respiratory tract. Study of the pattern of deposition of particles along the airways and the development of

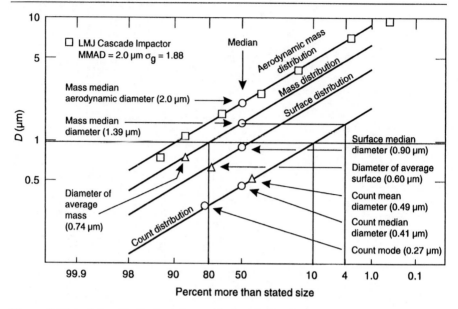

Figure 8. Plot of size distribution of an aerosol on log-probability paper. Curves are shown which characterize aerosol size in regard to various parameters

mathematical models to predict deposition has been continuous since the work of Findeisen.[15] Findeisen devised a model of the lung consisting of a regularly, dichotomously branching series of tubes divided into nine compartments, the last (representing the alveoli) numbering 5×10^7. He considered the pattern of deposition of spheres ranging in size from 0.03 to 30 μm in diameter. A simple model of the respiratory cycle was also used.[16] The model predicted complete deposition of spheres of diameter greater than 3 μm, a minimum of deposition (in fact about 35%) for spheres of diameter 0.1–0.3 μm, and a high total deposition for very small particles. Findeisen was working in a new field; he quoted only two references in his paper, both by Albert Einstein.

More complex mathematical models have been constructed by Landahl,[17] Hatch and Hemeon[18] and Altshuler.[19] Though the mathematical sophistication of the modelling has increased, the assumptions made regarding pulmonary anatomy have remained fairly simplistic.

A number of well-known graphs have been drawn to illustrate the predicted deposition of particles of different size in the respiratory tract. Figure 9 is taken from Muir,[2] and shows peak alveolar deposition at between 1 and 5 μm diameter.

Interest in particle deposition after World War II was fuelled by concern about possible deposition of radioactive particles. In 1965, The International Radiological Protection Commission (IRPC) Task Force on Lung Dynamics submitted its report: 'Deposition and retention models for internal dosimetry of the human respiratory

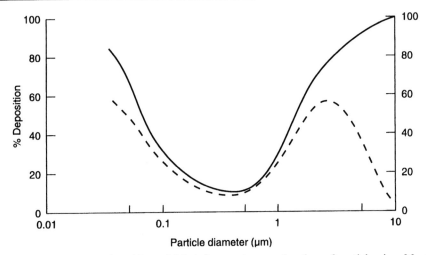

Figure 9. Percentage deposition of inhaled aerosols as a function of particle size. Mouth breathing at rest. Total deposition (—), alveolar deposition (— —). Reproduced with permission from DCF Muir (ed.) (1972) *Clinical Aspects of Inhaled Particles.* William Heinemann Books

tract.'[20] The Task Force, comprising Bates, Fish, Hatch, Mercer and Morrow, undertook a detailed examination of the area and developed a deposition model using methods of calculation similar to those used by Findeisen. The model was, however, more refined in terms of physiological parameters than that used by Findeisen. The respiratory tract was divided into three zones: nasopharyngeal (NP), tracheobronchial (TB) and pulmonary (P). The results of the deposition calculations for a range of particle sizes are shown in Table 8.

The pattern of deposition expected at a respiratory rate of 15 breaths per minute and a tidal volume of 750 ml is shown in Figure 10.

The effect of hygroscopic growth of particles was considered by the Task Force and is considered in detail below.

Having predicted the deposition of particles of different sizes, the Task Force calculated the predicted pattern of deposition of particles from polydisperse aerosols of known count median diameter and σ_g. The results of these most important calculations are shown in Table 9. The importance of this table cannot be overestimated: not so much because the predictions should be regarded as immutable, but because of the insight it provides into the factors controlling the deposition of particles in the respiratory tract. The data are plotted in Figure 11.

Figure 12 clearly illustrates minimal overall deposition of particles of 0.1–1.0 μm diameter. (In Figure 12, activity median aerodynamic diameter (relevant to radioactive particles) has been plotted.)

The models described above and more recent models based upon more realistic anatomical models of the respiratory tract[21-23] are based upon the calculations of the

Table 8. Deposition of unit density spheres

Tidal volume	Location	Diameter of sphere (μm)									
		0.01	0.06	0.20	0.60	1.0	2.0	3.0	4.0	6.0	10.0
750 cm³	N-P	0	0	0	0	0.036	0.406	0.552	0.654	0.799	0.992
	T-B	0.307	0.068	0.027	0.020	0.027	0.051	0.071	0.084	0.091	0.007
	P	0.506	0.585	0.281	0.204	0.250	0.346	0.308	0.238	0.103	0.002
1450 cm³	N-P	0	0	0	0	0.275	0.522	0.665	0.773	0.923	1.00
	T-B	0.256	0.051	0.017	0.019	0.027	0.050	0.064	0.069	0.043	0
	P	0.676	0.711	0.334	0.215	0.242	0.330	0.250	0.150	0.033	0
2150 cm³	N-P	0	0	0	0.068	0.371	0.607	0.736	0.844	1.0	1.0
	T-B	0.208	0.035	0.015	0.021	0.030	0.056	0.067	0.062	0	0
	P	0.746	0.653	0.294	0.209	0.226	0.285	0.195	0.092	0	0

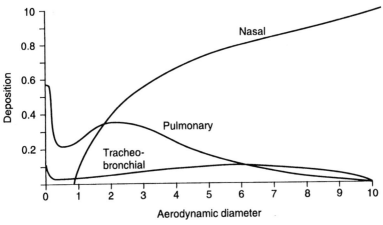

Figure 10. Deposition as a function of particle size for 15 respirations per minute, 750 cm^3 tidal volume. Reproduced with permission from Task Group on Lung Dynamics (1966) Deposition and retention models for internal dosimetry of the human respiratory tract. *Health Physics*, **12**, 173–207. © Williams & Wilkins

Table 9. Computed deposition of log-normal aerosols

MMAD (μm)	CMAD (μm)	Sigma (σ_g)	N-P	T-B	P
			\multicolumn{3}{c}{(per cent of inspired dust)}		
0.020	0.018	1.2	0.00	21.3	68.3
0.020	0.012	1.5	0.00	19.7	65.4
0.020	0.005	2.0	5.20*	20.7*	62.7*
0.020	0.002	2.5	6.70*	22.1*	59.0*
0.20	0.181	1.2	0.00	2.06	36.4
0.20	0.122	1.5	0.01	2.37	39.1
0.20	0.047	2.0	0.78	2.91	41.2
0.20	0.016	2.5	2.36	3.61	42.3
0.20	0.005	3.0	4.09	4.24	42.8
2.00	1.221	1.5	51.1	4.70	27.2
2.00	0.473	2.0	50.7	4.30	23.6
2.00	0.161	2.5	50.4	3.90	21.8
2.00	0.054	3.0	50.2	3.61	21.0
2.00	0.006	4.0	50.1	3.30	20.6
20.0	18.10	1.2	99.9	0.00	0.00
20.0	1.611	2.5	97.2	0.81	1.70
20.0	0.535	3.0	95.6	1.03	2.60
200.0	181.0	1.2	86.0	0.00	0.00

* Aerosol mass below 0.01 μm is presumed to experience an equal deposition in the three compartments: this is an estimated division reflecting the increased deposition probabilities of very small particles in the airways.
Reproduced with permission from Task Group on Lung Dynamics (1966) Deposition and retention models for internal dosimetry of the human respiratory tract. *Health Physics*, **12**, 173–207. © Williams & Wilkins.

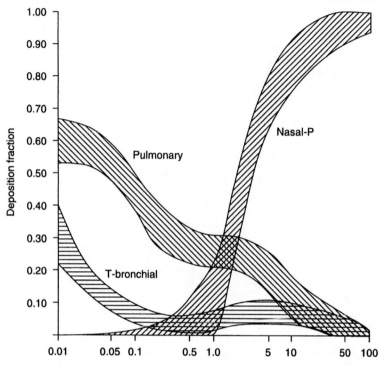

Figure 11. Shaded areas indicate variability of deposition for a given mass median (aerodynamic) diameter in each compartment when the distribution parameter, σ_g, varies from 1.2 to 4.5, and tidal volume is 1450 ml. Reproduced with permission from DCF Muir (ed.) (1972) *Clinical Aspects of Inhaled Particles*. William Heinemann Books

relative importance of a number of mechanisms of particle deposition. These are discussed in the following section.

MECHANISMS OF PARTICLE DEPOSITION

Sedimentation

Particles of density (ρ_{part}) greater than that of air (ρ_{air}) sediment under the force of gravity. As particles fall they accelerate until the resistive forces due to motion through the air equal the force applied by gravity. Once this occurs, the particle continues to fall at a constant velocity: the terminal velocity. Terminal velocity (V_t) may be calculated as follows.

Stokes[4] showed that the force exerted by gravity upon a falling body could be given by:

$$F_g = \frac{4}{3}\pi r^3(\rho_{part} - \rho_{air})g$$

where r is the radius of the particle, and g is the acceleration due to gravity.

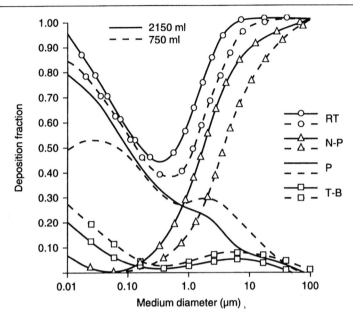

Figure 12. Two ventilatory states, i.e. 750 ml and 2150 ml tidal volume ($\sim$ 11 and $\sim$ 32 l min^{-1} volumes, respectively), are used to indicate the order and direction of change in compartmental deposition which are induced by such physiological factors. Note the cross-over in the 'P' curves at approximately 0.8 μm diameter (AMAD). Reproduced with permission from Task Group on Lung Dynamics (1966) Deposition and retention models for internal dosimetry of the human respiratory tract. *Health Physics*, **12**, 173–207. © Williams & Wilkins

He also showed that the resistive forces due to the motion of the body through the air could be given by:

$$F_{res} = 6\pi\eta r V$$

where η is the coefficient of viscosity of air and v is the velocity of the body.

For small particles where particle diameter is similar to the mean free path of gas molecules (λ), Cunningham's correction factor C_c must be applied:

$$F_{res} = \frac{6\pi\eta r V}{C_c}$$

When $F_g = F_{res}$ then the particle will have reached its terminal velocity:

$$\frac{6\pi\eta V_t}{C_c} = \frac{4}{3}\pi r^3 (\rho_{part} - \rho_{air})g$$

$$V_t = \frac{4}{3}\pi r^3 \frac{C_c}{6\pi\eta r}(\rho_{part} - \rho_{air})g$$

$$V_t = \frac{4}{18\eta}r^2 C_c(\rho_{part} - \rho_{air})g$$

Note that V_t or rate of sedimentation is proportional to the square of the radius of the particle.

Let

$$d = \text{particle diameter}$$
$$d = 2r$$
$$d^2 = 4r^2$$
$$r^2 = d^2/4$$

Then:

$$V_t = (\rho_{\text{part}} - \rho_{\text{air}}) \frac{C_c g d^2}{18\eta}$$

Cunningham's correction factor is given by:

$$C_c = 1 + 2.52 \frac{\lambda}{d}$$

Valberg stated that the equation for terminal velocity quoted above was valid for particles of unit density of diameter 0.1–40 μm, settling in air.[24] Correction factors allowing predictions to be made for particles of 0.001–200 μm diameter have been provided by Davies.[25]

Impaction

If the airstream in which a particle is travelling suddenly changes direction, e.g. at the bifurcation of an airway, force will be applied to the particle, causing it to move across the airstream. Should the particle encounter the wall of the tube in which the air is flowing during its journey across the stream, it will be deposited by impaction. Of course, the particle does not move at right angles across the stream, but follows a curved trajectory. If the particle was initially at the centre of the stream then it would come to rest (with regard to the direction of flow of the airstream), assuming it had not impacted on a wall, at some distance away from the centre of the stream, and continue along with the stream in this new position. The distance travelled (χ) before the particle comes to rest with regard to the airstream is given by Valberg[24] by:

$$\chi = \left(\frac{u \sin \theta}{g} \right) V_t$$

where u is velocity before deflection and θ is the angle of deflection of the airstream. V_t is the terminal velocity of the particle as calculated above. Note that here again, the deposition is dependent upon V_t and hence upon the square of the diameter (or radius) of the particle. Valberg[24] calculated that a sphere of unit density and 1.0 μm diameter travelling in an airstream at 1 m s^{-1} (typical of velocity in a major bronchus) would move 1.7 μm away from its previous stream line when the direction of airflow changed by 30°. This is a small movement. Deposition of particles in the airways as a result of impaction relates to those particles close to the walls of the airway, is proportional to the square of the particle radius and will be most efficient at bifurcations of the airways.

Impaction will also be most effective as a means of particle deposition when air velocity is high. As air moves down the respiratory tract, airflow velocity falls: impaction is most important in the larger airways. The effect of falling velocity of airflow is, as pointed out by Muir,[2] offset to some extent by the reduction in airway diameter: 'the fraction of particles entering the tenth generation of airways removed by impaction is similar to that removed in the third generation'.

The phenomenon of impaction has been thoroughly analysed both theoretically and experimentally and forms the basis of one of the most commonly used methods of particle sizing. Hinds' account of impactors should be consulted for details.[11] In essence, impactors direct a jet of particle-containing air via a nozzle towards a plate. The plate causes a 90° change in direction of flow, and some particles will impact upon the plate. Control of flow rate and nozzle diameter allows size control of the particles deposited.

Diffusion

The molecules of a gas are in constant motion and collide with aerosol particles. If these particles are small they are disturbed by the impact of the gas molecules and move in an irregular fashion described as Brownian motion. Particles moving in this way may encounter the walls of the airways and thus be deposited. The root mean square displacement after time t is given by:

$$\Delta = \sqrt{6Dt}$$

where D is the diffusion coefficient of the particle, and is given by:

$$D = \frac{KTC_c}{3\pi\eta d}$$

where T is the absolute temperature, K the Boltzmann constant, η the gas viscosity, C_c the Cunningham correction factor, and d the diameter of the particle. It should be noted that the smaller the particle, the greater will be the displacement in a given period.

Valberg[24] presented a useful table comparing displacement due to Brownian motion and that due to sedimentation (Table 10). The table makes clear that for very small particles diffusion will be the more important mechanism of deposition.

Interception

Interception occurs when long fibres travelling in the airstream impact upon airway walls as a result of not being able to bend with changes in direction of airflow. It is

Table 10. Root mean square Brownian displacement in 1 s compared with distance fallen in air in 1 s of unit density particles of different diameter

	Diameter (μm)	Brownian displacement in 1 s (μm)	Distance fallen in 1 s (μm)
Settling greater in 1 s	50	1.7	70 000
	20	2.7	11 500
	10	3.8	2 900
	5	5.5	740
	2	8.8	125
	1	13.0	33
Diffusion greater in 1 s	0.5	20	9.5
	0.2	37	2.1
	0.1	64	0.81
	0.05	120	0.35
	0.02	290	0.013
	0.01	570	0.0063

Temperature 37°C; gas viscosity 1.9×10^{-5} Pa s. Appropriate correction factors were applied for motion outside the range of validity of Stokes' law.
Reproduced with permission from Valberg PA (1985) Determination of retained lung dose from toxicology of inhaled materials. In: *Handbook of Experimental Pharmacology*, Vol. 75 (HP Witschi and JD Brain, eds), pp. 57–91. Berlin: Springer-Verlag. © 1985 Springer-Verlag.

an important means of deposition of fibres of materials such as asbestos but is not important in a CW context.

Electrostatic precipitation

Particles and surfaces may be described as charged if an excess of negative or positive charges exists at their surface. Charged particles are attracted to surfaces which carry the opposite charge to that upon the particles. The lining of the airways is uncharged. 'Image charge' can be induced at the surface by the approach of a charged particle and deposition is enhanced in comparison with that of uncharged particles. Valberg pointed out that electrostatic effects were likely to be important if a particle carried more than 10 charges upon its surface.[24] Charged particles lose charge in the atmosphere and only in the case of 'highly charged, freshly generated particles' is deposition in the respiratory tract likely to be significantly dependent upon electrostatic precipitation.

In summary, there are a number of mechanisms by which particles are deposited in the respiratory tract. Impaction becomes less significant as one moves along the airways, sedimentation plays an increasingly important role and, in the terminal parts of the airway, diffusion of small particles is important.

HYGROSCOPIC GROWTH OF AND NEUTRALIZATION OF ACIDIC DROPLETS IN THE AIRWAYS

It was indicated above that particles or droplets (hereafter referred to as particles) of inorganic salts could grow in the airways as a result of condensation of water upon their surfaces. If particles were acidic or alkaline on inhalation, dilution with water will move the pH towards 7. In addition, ammonia, produced mainly by bacterial action in the mouth, is absorbed by particles and neutralization of acidic particles will occur.

Cocks and Fernando undertook a detailed theoretical analysis and computer simulation of the growth of droplets on passing from ambient air to the conditions obtaining in the lung.[6] Predicted patterns of growth are shown in Figure 13. The growth of particles of two initial sizes was modelled. Droplets of 0.1 and 1.0 μm radius containing 20%, 40% and 60% solutions of sulphuric acid were considered. These solutions have vapour pressures corresponding to different relative humidities: 88%, 57% and 16% respectively. The Kelvin effect was taken into account in calculating these equivalent relative humidities: thus the vapour pressure (measured at a plane surface) of a 20% solution of sulphuric acid would be less than that exerted by water vapour at a RH of 88% or, alternatively, a droplet of 20% sulphuric acid and radius 0.1 μm is stable at a RH of 88% because this represents a slightly

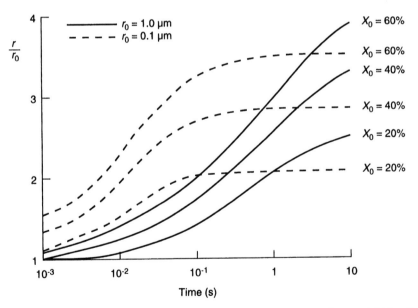

Figure 13. Growth curves for sulphuric acid droplets. r, equilibrium radius; r_0, initial radius; X_0, initial concentration of sulphuric acid. Reprinted from *Journal of Aerosol Science*, **13**, AT Cocks and RP Fernando, The growth of sulphate aerosols in the human airways, pp. 9–19, 1982, with kind permission from Elsevier Science Ltd, The Boulevard, Langford Lane, Kidlington OX5 1GB, UK

greater vapour pressure than would be exerted by 20% sulphuric acid at a plane surface.

It was assumed that the RH in the respiratory tract was 99.5%. It was discovered that smaller droplets would grow more rapidly than larger droplets and thus approached equilibrium size more rapidly. It was also noted that: 'comparing droplets of the same initial composition, those of smaller initial radii will attain a lower value of r/r_0 (equilibrium radius/initial radius) given sufficient time than larger droplets'. This is due to the greater significance of the Kelvin effect, which retards the growth of small droplets.

Figure 14 illustrates the need for precise knowledge regarding the RH in the respiratory tract when predicting particle growth. Droplets containing 20% sulphuric acid of 0.1 and 1.0 μm radius were modelled growing under conditions of differing RH. Note that at humidities of 99.5% and 99% all particles approach an equilibrium radius.

As small particles grow, their diffusion-dependent deposition in the peripheral lung becomes less efficient. Conversely, as large particles grow, their sedimentation and impaction-dependent deposition in the upper airways would be expected to increase. Thus the overall effect of hygroscopic growth on particle deposition in the respiratory tract may be difficult to predict: an effect on location of deposition might,

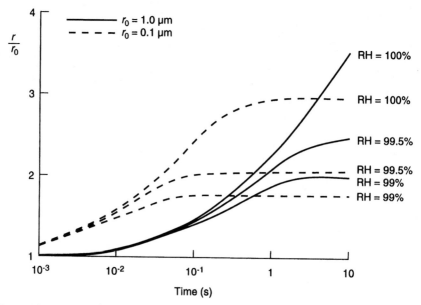

Figure 14. The effect of the assumed relative humidity in the lung on the growth of sulphuric acid droplets. r, equilibrium radius; r_0, initial radius. Reprinted from *Journal of Aerosol Science*, **13**, AT Cocks and RP Fernando, The growth of sulphate aerosols in the human airways, pp. 9–19, 1982, with kind permission from Elsevier Science Ltd, The Boulevard, Langford Lane, Kidlington OX5 1GB, UK

however, be expected. Martonen et al.[26] illustrated the size-dependent differential effect of particle growth on deposition; see Figure 15.

The figure shows mass deposition fraction plotted against the initial geometric particle size. Martonen argued that a critical particle size could be defined: D_c. For hygroscopic particles initially smaller than this size, hygroscopic growth would be expected to reduce deposition compared with that of non-hygroscopic particles. The extent of the reduction in deposition is shown for a particle of initial diameter 0.1 μm by AB. For hygroscopic particles of greater initial diameter than D_c hygroscopic growth would increase deposition: the effect on particles of 0.7 μm initial diameter is shown by ED for oral breathing and CD for nasal breathing. Note that more growth occurs during nasal breathing, the inspired air being better humidified.

The effects of hygroscopic growth upon the regional deposition of particles in the respiratory tract have been considered by Pritchard.[7] Figure 16 shows the shift in the deposition pattern of particles produced by hygroscopic growth. As might be expected, a shift to the right in the pattern of deposition is demonstrated. For hygroscopic particles, minimum deposition is associated with an initial particle diameter of 0.1 μm. For non-hygroscopic particles the size of minimum deposition

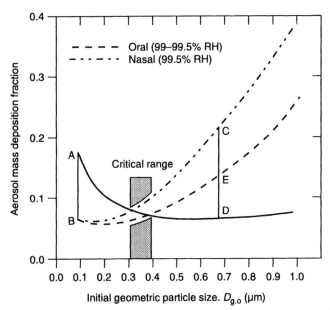

Figure 15. The influence of inhaled particle size and breathing mode on ammonium sulphate aerosol deposition: (—) non-hygroscopic particle behaviour included for comparison. Minute volume = 30 l. Reproduced with permission from Martonen TB (1985) Ambient sulphate deposition in man: modelling the influence of hygroscopicity. *Environmental Health Perspectives*, **63**, 11–24

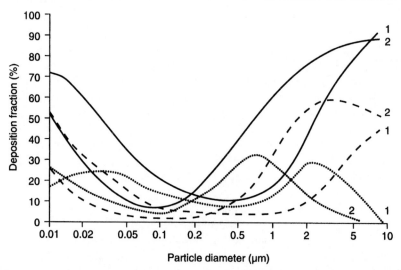

Figure 16. Total and regional distribution of hygroscopic particles in the lung. Oral breathing: tidal volume, 500 ml; breathing rate, 13.7 breaths per minutes. 1, non-hygroscopic; 2, hygroscopic. Solid line, total deposition; dotted line, deposition in pulmonary region; dashed line, deposition in tracheobronchial region. Reproduced from Pritchard JN (1987) Particle growth in the airways and the influence of airflow. In *A New Concept in Inhalation Therapy* (SP Newman, F Moren and GK Crompton, eds), Medicom

was closer to 0.5 μm. In these studies the hygroscopic particles considered were sodium chloride: such particles would show maximal hygroscopic growth which would not be matched by other particles.

The Task Group of IRPC considered the effects of particle growth upon likely deposition in the respiratory tract and pointed out that for particles of high density, hygroscopic growth would have less effect than might be predicted from a simple consideration of the effects of an increase in particle diameter.[20] Addition of water to a dense particle will reduce particle density and offset the effect of increasing real diameter on the aerodynamic diameter. The ratio of aerodynamic diameter of the particle after hygroscopic growth to that of the original dry particle is given by:

$$\frac{D_{AS}}{D_{AC}} = \left[\frac{\rho_s C_s}{\rho_c C_c}\right]^{\frac{1}{2}} \frac{D_s}{D_c}$$

where ρ_c and ρ_s are the densities of the dry particle and the droplet respectively, D_{AS} and D_{AC} are the aerodynamic diameters of the droplet and the original particle respectively, D_s and D_c are the actual diameters, and C_s and C_c are the respective Cunningham's correction factors.

It is clear that droplets may change their composition as they pass along the airways. Little work has been reported on this as regards effects on CW agents, but extensive and informative studies have been undertaken on acid droplets. Droplets of sulphuric acid grow as they pass along the airways. It has been calculated that a particle of less than 0.1 μm initial diameter would reach 99% of its equilibrium diameter on being exposed to the air of the respiratory tract for as little as 0.1 s. This should be compared with the 10 s needed for a droplet of 1.0 μm initial diameter to reach 99% of equilibrium diameter.

Consider a droplet of sulphuric acid growing in the airstream in the respiratory tract: assuming the equilibrium radius of a particle to be 3 times the initial radius, the equilibrium volume will be 27 times the initial volume. Given also that no sulphuric acid is added to the particle during growth, then the sulphuric acid concentration will fall during particle growth by a factor of 27.

Let the initial hydrogen ion molar concentration $= x_0$ M. Then:

$$\text{equilibrium hydrogen ion concentration} = x_0/27 \text{ M}$$
$$\text{Initial pH} = -\log x_0$$
$$\text{Equilibrium pH} = -\log x_0/27$$
$$= -(\log x_0 - \log 27)$$
$$= -\log x_0 + 1.4314$$

The dilution factor of 27 will increase the pH of the droplet by approximately 1.4.

NEUTRALIZATION OF ACID DROPLETS BY AMMONIA IN THE RESPIRATORY TRACT

Ammonia is produced in the mouth as a result of bacterial metabolism. Kupprat *et al.* measured ammonia concentrations of between 210 and 700 μg m^{-3} in expired air during quiet mouth breathing.[27] Larson recorded values of 10–50 μg m^{-3} during quiet nasal breathing.[28]

Acid droplets absorb ammonia and become partially neutralized as they pass along the respiratory tract. Cocks and McElroy[29] extended the work already discussed[6] on the hygroscopic growth of particles to model the growth and neutralization of acid aerosols. Before considering the results of the Cocks and McElroy study,[29] two difficulties identified and dealt with by these authors should be examined:

1. One might ask whether droplets of sulphuric acid which have been neutralized by ammonia and converted into droplets of a solution of ammonium sulphate would grow hygroscopically at the same rate as the original droplets of acid. Cocks and Fernando[6] modelled the growth of droplets of ammonium bisulphate and ammonium sulphate and showed that the expected growth patterns were very similar to that of sulphuric acid droplets. The results of this modelling exercise are shown in Figure 17.

2. Acid aerosols are often found in association with high concentrations of acidic gases such as sulphur dioxide. It might, therefore, be asked whether significant depletion of nasal or oral ammonia by sulphur dioxide might occur and thus impair droplet neutralization. This was modelled by Cocks and McElroy,[29] who

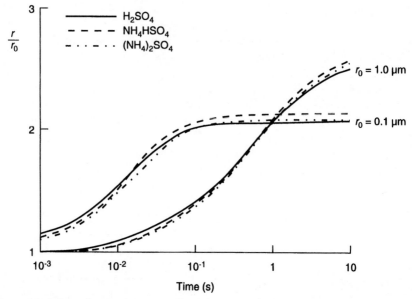

Figure 17. Effect of neutralization by ammonia on the growth of sulphuric acid droplets. r, equilibrium radius; r_0, initial radius. Reprinted from *Journal of Aerosol Science*, **13**, AT Cocks and RP Fernando, The growth of sulphate aerosols in the human airways, pp. 9–19, 1982, with kind permission from Elsevier Science Ltd, The Boulevard, Langford Lane, Kidlington OX5 1GB, UK

concluded that at a sulphur dioxide concentration of 100 μg m^{-3} only some 2% of the ammonia likely to be present would be removed in 10 s. The effect may be neglected.

In the main modelling exercise Cocks and McElroy[29] modelled the following.

Acid loading of the atmosphere: 1000 and 100 μg m^{-3}

It should be noted that given constant relative humidity and all the acid being assumed to be contained in droplets of a given size, e.g. 0.1 μm diameter, there will be 10 times as many droplets present per unit volume of air at the higher loading than at the lower loading.

Ammonia concentration

These were 500 μg m^{-3} corresponding to oral levels and 50 μg m^{-3} corresponding to nasal levels.

Initial droplet composition

As explained earlier, droplets of sulphuric acid of differing size and acid

Table 11. Sulphuric acid concentrations in stable droplets at varying ambient relative humidity

RH (%)	$[H_2SO_4]$ M
99.97	7.0×10^{-3}
99.5	0.139
80	3.29
60	5.08

concentration are in stable equilibrium at different relative humidities. The authors calculated that acid concentration and RH under conditions of stable equilibrium were related as shown in Table 11.

Let us assume that all the acid is present in 5-μm-diameter droplets.

Let us also assume that the acid loading of the air is 1000 μg m^{-3}.

Now consider a relative humidity of 99.97%. The droplets will contain acid at a concentration of 7×10^{-3} M.

Now consider a relative humidity of 60%. The droplets will contain acid at a concentration of 5.08 M.

In both cases total acid loading is constant. This could only be accomplished if there were many more droplets present per unit volume of air at a relative humidity of 99.97% as compared with air at a relative humidity of 60%.

The ratio of the number of droplets present in the two cases is given by:

$$(5.08/7) \times 10^{-3} = 725.7$$

That is, at an atmospheric loading of X μg m^{-3} with the acid contained in droplets of diameter y μm, there will be 725.7 times as many droplets present in unit volume of air at a relative humidity of 99.97% than at 60%.

Initial droplet diameter

Diameters of 0.1, 0.5, 5.0 and 15 μm were considered. Not all droplet diameters were modelled for each value of relative humidity.

The following were calculated for 0.1, 0.3, 1.0, 3.0 and 10 s of growth.

Reduction in droplet acidity (H)

$$H = [H^+]/[H^+]_0$$

Extent of neutralization (N) expressed as a percentage

$$N = [NH_4^+]/(2([HSO_4^-] + [SO_4^{2-}])) \times 100$$

Complete neutralization is reached when $[NH_4^+]$ is twice the concentration of sulphur(VI)-containing molecules. This is complex: it may be approached as follows.

When ammonia in solution reacts with sulphuric acid: two NH_4^+ ions are produced for each SO_4^{2-} ion, one NH_4^+ ion is produced for each HSO_4^- ion and a further NH_4^+ ion is produced in converting the acidic HSO_4^- ion to a neutral SO_4^{2-} ion.

Neutrality is reached when the concentration of NH_4^+ ions is twice the sum of the concentrations of the SO_4^{2-} ions and the HSO_4^- ions, i.e.

$$[NH_4^+] = 2([HSO_4^-] + [SO_4^{2-}])$$

The contribution of droplet growth to the change in acidity (V)

$$V = V_0/V$$

It will be appreciated that a complex matrix of results was generated by this modelling exercise. From the detailed tables of results presented by the authors, certain particularly interesting results have been selected for more detailed consideration here.

For the results shown in Table 12, the model has included sufficient ammonia to bring about complete neutralization of the acid droplets in the air. As the initial relative humidity was high (99.5%), no hygroscopic growth of the particles occurred. Complete neutralization of 5-μm droplets would be expected in 3 s. The capacity of the ammonia present to neutralize all the acid present should be contrasted with the extent of neutralization possible had the ammonia concentration been 50 μg m^{-3}.

Calculation of the extent of neutralization possible given an acid loading of 1000 μg m^{-3} and an ammonia concentration of 50 μg m^{-3}.

$\underline{H_2SO_4:}$ $\underline{GMW = 98\ g}$ $\underline{NH_3:}$ $\underline{GMW = 17\ g}$

$1\ \mu g = 1/98 \times 10^{-6}\ M$

$\qquad = 2/98 \times 10^{-6}\ Eq$

$1000\ \mu g = 2/98 \times 10^{-6} \times 10^3\ Eq \qquad\qquad 50\ \mu g = 1/17 \times 10^{-6} \times 50\ Eq$

$\qquad \approx 20 \times 10^{-6}\ Eq \qquad\qquad\qquad\qquad = 2.94 \times 10^{-6}\ Eq$

Neutralization ratio $= 2.94/20 = 0.147 = 14.7\%$

The results shown in Table 12 should be compared with those in Table 13. Here, again, no hygroscopic growth occurred but neutralization was very rapid as a result of the high surface to volume ratio of the small droplets.

The results shown in Table 14 are more difficult to interpret. Neutralization is slow because of the high acid content of each droplet. However, considerable hygroscopic growth occurs and droplet acidity is more affected by droplet growth than by droplet

Table 12. Data from the Cocks–McElroy model of droplet growth and neutralization

$[H_2SO_4]$ ($\mu g\ m^{-3}$)	$[NH_3]$ ($\mu g\ m^{-3}$)	Droplet diameter (μm)		Time (s)				
				0.1	0.3	1	3	10
1000	500	5	H	0.822	0.535	0.087	5.2×10^{-4}	
RH = 99.5%			V	1.0	1.0	1.0	1.0	
$[H_2SO_4]_0 = 0.139$ M			N	11.7	32.3	81.9	100	

neutralization. It should be noted that acidity has fallen to 40% of its original value by 0.1 s despite the fact that neutralization has only reached 0.42%.

For Table 15, the same conditions as shown in Table 14 are simulated except that the initial droplet diameter is set at 1.0 μm. Here the droplets are neutralized more rapidly as a result of the more favourable surface to volume ratio and also grow more rapidly than the 5-μm droplets. Almost complete neutralization and reduction of droplet acid concentration to low levels is achieved by 1.0 s.

These studies show clearly that substantial changes in size and composition of aerosol droplets may occur during passage along the respiratory tract. It is not surprising that hygroscopic growth may produce significant changes in patterns of deposition of particles. Interestingly, hygroscopic growth is in part dependent upon the pattern of airflow in the airway. This will be considered when the general effects of increased ventilation upon particle deposition have been considered.

Muir[2] reviewed the effects of variations in the pattern of breathing upon total particle deposition and on the distribution of the deposited particles along the respiratory tract: the effects are complex. Inertial deposition of particles is dependent upon the velocity of the particles and hence upon the velocity of the airstream. Sedimentation and diffusion-dependent deposition are dependent upon the time available for particle displacement to bring particles into contact with the walls of the airways. Deposition of large particles in the upper airways might be expected to rise under conditions of increased airflow. Increased rates of airflow increase the likelihood of turbulent flow occurring and this again increases the likelihood of particles on the walls of the airways. Turbulent flow occurs in the airways when Reynold's number exceeds about 1000. Muir summarized the effects of changing airflow as follows.

Table 13. Data from the Cocks–McElroy model of droplet growth and neutralization

$[H_2SO_4]$ ($\mu g\ m^{-3}$)	$[NH_3]$ ($\mu g\ m^{-3}$)	Droplet diameter (μm)		Time (s)				
				0.1	0.3	1	3	10
1000	500	1.0	H	5.2×10^{-4}				
RH = 99.5%			V	1.0				
$[H_2SO_4]_0 = 0.139$ M			N	100				

Table 14. Data from the Cocks–McElroy model of droplet growth and neutralization

[H$_2$SO$_4$] (μg m^{-3})	[NH$_3$] (μg m^{-3})	Droplet diameter (μm)		Time (s)				
				0.1	0.3	1	3	10
1000 RH = 60%	500	5	H	0.400	0.241	0.126	0.063	0.011
			V	0.398	0.241	0.134	0.081	0.048
[H$_2$SO$_4$]$_0$ = 5.08–5.17 M			N	0.42	1.43	5.43	19.0	61.5

For a given minute ventilation rapid shallow breathing reduces overall particle deposition and, in particular, reduces the fraction of the aerosol penetrating to the alveoli. On the other hand slow, deep, breathing increases the deposition of the aerosol in the depths of the lung . . . .

Muir went on to point out that during exercise minute volume increases as a result of increases in both tidal volume and breathing rate. Increases in tidal volume would lead to particles being drawn further into the lung and would offset the reduced fractional deposition which might be expected had only the respiratory rate increased. Muir and Davies confirmed, using 0.5 μm-diameter particles, that fractional deposition remained constant in the resting and exercising subject.[30] Dennis in a study using larger particles (1.0–3.0 μm diameter) showed an increase in the deposition fraction with minute volume.[31] Given that the deposition fraction does not fall during exercise, it follows that total particle deposition will increase with minute volume.

During exercise, oral breathing becomes increasingly important and the reduction in fractional deposition in the nose will increase the fraction of the inspired aerosol delivered to the lung.

Pritchard has drawn attention to the increased rate of removal of latent heat from particles undergoing hygroscopic growth under conditions of turbulent airflow.[7] As growth rate is dependent upon the rate of removal of latent heat, conditions of turbulent flow increase hygroscopic growth rates. Given that inertial impaction is dependent upon the square of particle diameter, increased hygroscopic growth will increase particle deposition. Of course, this effect may be offset in the upper airways by the reduced particle residence time imposed by increased flow rates: deposition in

Table 15. Data from the Cocks–McElroy model of droplet growth and neutralization

[H$_2$SO$_4$] (μg m^{-3})	[NH$_3$] (μg m^{-3})	Droplet diameter (μm)		Time (s)				
				0.1	0.3	1	3	10
1000 RH = 60%	500	1.0	H	0.09	0.028	2.9 $\times$ 10^{-5}	2.0 $\times$ 10^{-5}	1.8 $\times$ 10^{-5}
			V	0.115	0.07	0.043	0.032	0.029
[H$_2$SO$_4$]$_0$ = 5.08–5.17 M			N	14.3	44.6	99.9	99.9	99.9

the smaller airways would then be likely to be increased. Pritchard,[7] using data from Martonen,[26] produced Table 16. The significant effects are illustrated by comparison of the sets of figures printed in bold typeface. The marked increase in deposition of 1.0-μm particles in the upper airway under conditions of nasal breathing and high flow rate is obvious. Interestingly, the fractional deposition ratio between upper and lower airways is reversed under these conditions as compared with low-flow-rate nasal breathing.

GENERAL CONCEPTS CONCERNING THE TOXICITY OF CW AGENTS

The toxicity of a compound may be defined in a number of ways. The descriptor until recently used in general toxicology and still widely used when thinking about CW agents is the LD_{50}. This specifies the dose of the compound in question which would be expected to kill 50% of a group of animals of the same species, i.e. the median lethal dose. The statement 'the LD_{50} of lewisite is 2 mg kg^{-1}' is, as it stands, meaningless. Only when the route of administration and the species are specified does the statement become informative. Computer-stored toxicology databases often list LD_{50} data with the essential qualifications added, e.g.

$$\text{lewisite, } LD_{50} \text{ (subcut, dog)} = 2 \text{ mg kg}^{-1}$$

LD_{50} values are derived from a study of the toxicity of the given compound. This involves exposing groups of animals to different doses of the test compound and

Table 16. The influence of breathing pattern on ammonium bisulphate deposition in the lung

	Flow = 15 l min^{-1} Particle size			Flow = 60 l min^{-1} Particle size		
	0.1 μm	0.5 μm	1.0 μm	0.1 μm	0.5 μm	1.0 μm
Deposition under oral breathing %						
Region: Upper	0	1	2	0	2	8
Middle	2	2	5	1	4	14
Lower	7	8	21	4	6	12
Total	9	11	28	5	12	34
Deposition under nasal breathing %						
Region: Upper	0	2	**7**	0	8	**30**
Middle	2	3	**8**	1	7	**16**
Lower	7	8	**19**	4	5	**19**
Total	9	13	**34**	5	20	**65**

Upper region: airway generation 0–5
Middle region: airway generation 6–10
Lower region: airway generation 11–15
Reproduced from Pritchard JN (1987) Particle growth in the airways and the influence of airflow. In *A New Concept in Inhalation Therapy* (SP Newman, F Moren and GK Crompton, eds). Medicom.

noting the incidence of deaths in the groups by a given time. Hence a further refinement is added to the LD_{50}: the time at which the count of decedents was made. This should be added to the statement of the LD_{50}.

The LD_{50} may be derived graphically from a plot of the probit transform of the incidence of death against the logarithm of the dose administered. This is the classical quantal assay.

The basis of the probit transform lies in the observation that, for a wide range of toxic compounds, if the incidence of mortality is plotted against the logarithm of the dose of the test compound the distribution curve obtained approximates to the cumulative normal distribution curve. As the steps taken in moving from this observation to the 'probit slope' are a little complicated, an example, starting with hypothetical data and working through to the probit slope, is given below.

Consider the hypothetical data given in Table 17. These data may be plotted in a number of ways. If the percentage mortality is plotted against dose the curve shown in Figure 18 is obtained. If the percentage mortality is plotted against log dose, the curve shown in Figure 19 is obtained. This conforms closely to a cumulative normal distribution curve.

To understand the next manipulation the normal distribution curve should be recalled (Figure 20). The probability of an observation falling between any two values of x may be described by the proportion of the whole area under the curve occupied by the area bounded by the two values. For example, the probability that

Table 17. Hypothetical data relating dose to mortality

Dose d_i	Log (dose)	Mortality m_i			Tolerance $m_i - m_{i-1}$ (%)
		Obs	(%)	Probit	
0.3	−0.3	0/40	0	—	0
1.0	0.0	1/40	2.5	3.04	2.5
1.5	0.176	4/410	10	3.72	7.5
2.0	0.3	9/40	22.5	4.24	12.5
2.5	0.4	15/40	37.5	4.68	15
3.0	0.48	21/40	52.5	5.06	15
3.5	0.54	25/40	62.5	5.32	10
4.0	0.60	29/40	72.5	5.60	10
4.5	0.65	32/40	80	5.84	7.5
5.0	0.70	34/40	85	6.04	5
5.5	0.74	36/40	90	6.28	5
6.0	0.78	37/40	92.5	6.44	2.5
6.5	0.81	38/40	95	6.64	2.5
7.0	0.85	39/40	97.5	6.96	2.5
7.5	0.88	40/40	100	—	2.5

d = dose.
d_i = i'th dose.
m = mortality.
m_i = mortality at the i'th dose.

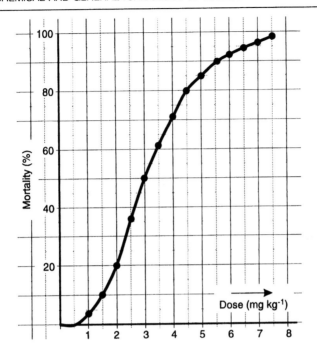

Figure 18. Data from Table 17 plotted arithmetically

measurements of x will fall between a and b in Figure 20 is given by the proportion of the whole area under the curve occupied by the shaded area. This may, of course, be thought of in terms of the standard deviation: 68.2% of observations fall within $+1$ and -1 standard deviations of the mean; in fact, a and b in Figure 20 are standard deviations. Ninety-five per cent of observations lie between $+1.96$ and -1.96 SDs, and 99% of observations lie between $+3$ and -3 SDs of the mean. Intermediate values may be obtained from statistical tables of the normal distribution curve.

The scale along the x-axis of Figure 20, in units of standard deviation, i.e.

$$\frac{x - \bar{x}}{\text{SD}}$$

is described as the scale of normal equivalent deviation and the values -3, -2, -1, 0, $+1$, $+2$, $+3$ are called NEDs or normal equivalent deviates. If 5 is added to each value of the NED, the equivalent 'probit' values are obtained. Finney[32] commented on the origin of these terms: 'Bliss (1934) first proposed the name "probit" for his modification of Gaddum's normal equivalent deviate [NED], which he increased by 5 so as to simplify the arithmetical procedure by avoiding negative values.' Probabilities for NED > 5 are seldom encountered: NED $= -5$ is equivalent to about 1 in a million. Table 18 shows the equivalence between NEDs and probits.

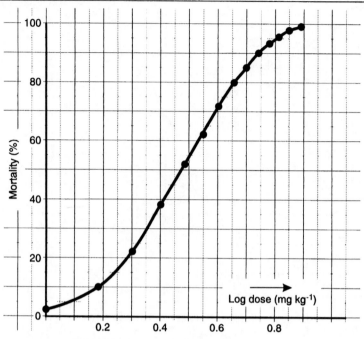

Figure 19. Data from Table 17 plotted using the log of the dose. This could have been shown on semi-log paper by simply plotting the dose on the x-axis

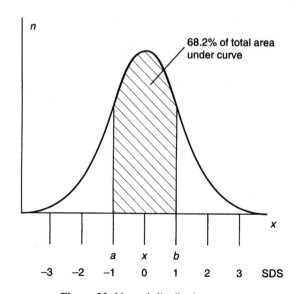

Figure 20. Normal distribution curve

Recalling how the percentage of observations lay on the normal distribution curve in terms of NEDs allows one to deduce how they will lie in terms of probits. This is shown in Figure 21.

More accurate calculation of probits from the equation of the normal distribution curve has been undertaken and tables are available.

If instead of percentage mortality the corresponding probits are plotted against log dose, a straight line is obtained (Figure 22). The median lethal dose, i.e. the dose at which 50% of the animals would be expected to die, may simply be read off the graph. In practice the actual dose is plotted on a logarithmic scale on the x-axis and the percentage mortality on the y-axis on a scale modified so as to correspond to the probit scale. Such special graph paper is described as log-probability paper, which has been mentioned before in this chapter, and is widely used in toxicology. Figure 23 shows the same data as discussed above plotted on this paper.

A question often asked by students of toxicology is: 'Why does the probit versus log dose plot so often come out as a straight line?' This remarkably simple question is difficult to answer. It may be approached in two stages.

Given that a log-normal distribution curve may be used to describe the relationship regarding tolerance of the species in question to compound x, then the probit–log dose plot must yield a straight line. This is because the probit scale is related to the percentage mortality scale (i.e. the scale on the y-axis) in precisely the same way as the percentage mortality is related to the log dose (i.e. the scale on the x-axis).

This may be summarized:

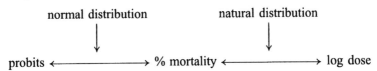

It is no surprise, then, that probits, which are derived from percentage mortality via the normal distribution curve, and log dose, which is related to percentage mortality by the normal distribution curve, should be related by a straight line.

An algebraic analogy may help:

Let $x = k \log y$: a non-linear relationship
Let $z = k' \log y$: a similar non-linear relationship
Then $x/z = k \log y / k' \log y$
$x = k/k'z$: a linear relationship

Table 18. Relationships between NEDs and probits

NEDs	− 3	− 2	− 1	0	1	2	3
Probits	2	3	4	5	6	7	8

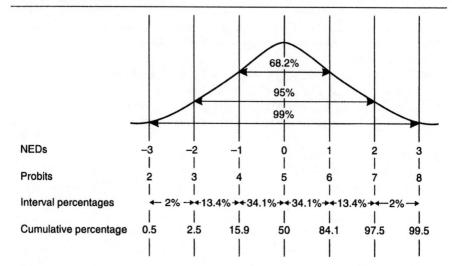

Figure 21. Normal distribution curve showing relationships between NEDs, probits and areas under the curve

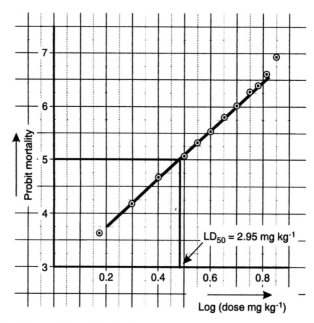

Figure 22. Data from Table 17 plotted showing the log of dose on the x-axis and the mortality probit on the y-axis.

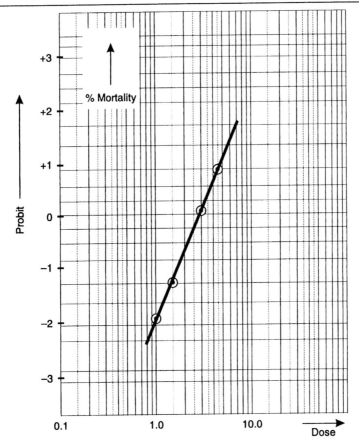

Figure 23. Data from Table 17 plotted on 'log-probability' paper

The second part of the explanation is much less satisfactory: why percentage mortality is related to log dose via the normal distribution curve is unknown.

Many CW agents are encountered as gases. Establishing the dose of a gas is difficult compared with that provided by, say, an intravenous injection. This has led to the definition of exposure rather than dose and to the concentration $\times$ time product. Exposure may be thus measured in terms of

$$\text{concentration (mg m}^{-3}) \times \text{duration of exposure (min)}$$

and the median lethal exposure determined experimentally as the LCt_{50}.

The units of Ct are mg m^{-3} min or, more euphorically but less obviously, mg min m^{-3}. The toxicity of the nerve agent sarin in humans is often given as 100 mg min m^{-3}.

The fundamental difference between LD_{50} and LCt_{50} is that the former relates to dose and the latter to exposure. It cannot be stressed too strongly: *exposure does not equal dose.*

In addition to the descriptors already identified for use with the LD_{50} value, species and time at which decedents are counted, another must be added regarding LCt_{50} (route need not normally be considered: LCt_{50} usually refers to inhalation, though in experimental studies absorption across the skin might be being studied).

A further additional factor describing the physiological conditions associated with the LCt_{50} must also be added. For example, sarin (GB) is well absorbed across the lung and some 90% of inhaled GB is absorbed. This is effectively independent of respiratory rate and depth. Thus a person breathing 50 l min^{-1} will take in five times as much GB as a person breathing 10 l min^{-1}. Thus, in an identical exposure, the dose absorbed by the former will be five times that absorbed by the latter. In terms of dose, the same dose will be inhaled by an exercising man though he is exposed, for the same period, to only one-fifth of the concentration of GB as a non-exercising man. Thus the LCt_{50} exercising $= 1/5 LCt_{50}$ at rest.

For GB:

$$\text{Human } LCt_{50} \text{ resting} = 100 \text{ mg min m}^{-3}$$

$$\text{Human } LCt_{50} \text{ exercising} = 20 \text{ mg min m}^{-3}$$

One more complicating factor must now be considered: the effect of duration of exposure. Consider the data shown in Table 19. In each of the rows the Ct product $= 100$ mg min m^{-3}. In the rows c, d and e one might feel reasonably confident that the mortality likely to occur would be about 50%, i.e. an LCt_{50} exposure. At the outer rows, one becomes distinctly less confident and it is unlikely that continuous exposure of a person to 0.0001 mg m^{-3} GB for 1.9 years would

Table 19. Toxicity of the nerve agent sarin (GB)

	C (mg m^{-3})	t (min)	Ct (mg min m^{-3})	Expected % mortality
a	10 000	0.01	100	?
b	1 000	0.1	100	? < 50
c	100	1	100	50
d	10	10	100	50
e	1	100	100	50
f	0.1	1 000	100	? < 50
g	0.01	10 000	100	?
h	0.001	100 000	100	?
i	0.0001	1 000 000	100	?

The values shown in lines c, d and e are approximately correct. Data in other lines have been derived on the assumption that the LCt is constant; this assumption is discussed in the text.

have the same effect as exposure to 10 mg m^{-3} for 10 min. Interestingly, the US permissible exposure limit for GB (expressed as an 8-h time weighted average, TWA), is 0.0001 mg m^{-3}: such an exposure, on a daily, life-long basis, would be regarded as safe.

The concept that a constant Ct product might be expected to produce a constant effect was propounded by F. Haber, who defined:

$$Ct = W$$

where W is 'product of mortality' (Todlichkeitsprodukt) or 'lethal index'.

The Haber relationship may be represented by a hyperbola. During World War I it was found that the toxicity of many CW agents deviated from the relationship proposed by Haber, and attempts to refine the real relationship were made. The equation:

$$(C - e) \times t = W$$

takes into account elimination (e) of the compound by metabolic processes.

One of the most interesting examples of deviations from the Haber relationship is provided by hydrogen cyanide. Consider the data in Table 20. At low concentrations the body is able to metabolize cyanide, and thus as long as the concentration is low a substantial total exposure may be tolerated. The LCt_{50} rises with the duration of exposure. This increase in LCt_{50}, with time, is intuitively understandable and fairly common; the converse, a fall of LCt_{50} with time, is rare but may occur.

Because of the ease of assessing lethality, many toxicity studies have concentrated upon determination of LD_{50} or LCt_{50}. Of more importance in the military context are the incapacitating effects of compounds, and the ID_{50} (median incapacitating dose) or the ICt_{50} are important descriptors of a compound's toxicity. These are of course much more difficult to determine in animals and the relevance of such determinations to likely effects in humans is open to doubt. Of even more military importance are the parameters ICt_5 and ICt_{10}, though to determine these with any accuracy is yet more difficult and great caution should be exercised when trying to determine these parameters from studies designed to identify the median exposures. The reliability of predictions made from the probit slope outside the $< 20\%$ to $> 80\%$ region is low.

Table 20. Relationship between duration of exposure (time) and concentration and LCt_{50} for hydrogen cyanide

Time (min)	Concentration (mg m^{-3})	LCt_{50} (mg min m^{-3})
0.25	2400	660
1.0	1000	1000
10	200	2000
15	133	4000

PARTICLES AS VECTORS FOR CHEMICAL WARFARE AGENTS

Since World War I, the suggestion that inert particles could be used as vectors for CW agents has recurred from time to time. Lefebure recorded that a prisoner of a German gas battalion had reported the use of small pumice granules impregnated with phosgene.[33] This was apparently an attempt to increase the persistence of phosgene under field conditions. Lefebure also considered that particulate clouds might penetrate respirators designed to absorb gases and, if combined with a lethal gas, present a significant threat. Much of the World War I development of arsenical smokes was based upon this concept. In part these ideas did not require the particles to act as vectors: a highly irritant particulate capable of penetrating the respirator and inducing coughing or vomiting would lead to removal of the respirator and possible exposure to a lethal compound such as phosgene. Attempts to develop particulate material impregnated with more or less volatile CW agents persisted into the 1930s and 1940s. Mustard-gas-impregnated dust was studied extensively in Germany in this period. Dautrebande,[34] commenting on the role of particles as vectors, noted:

> For example, when submitted to mustard gas vapours (25 mg/m^3 for 30 minutes) rats do not develop signs of general toxicity or of respiratory distress; simply, in the following days, they exhibit irritation of the accessible mucosae (eyes, nose, ears, rectum) and are all completely cured after three weeks. On the other hand, when submitted for the same length of time (30 minutes) to a concentration of vesicant vapours of 5 mg/m^3 only (instead of 25 mg/m^3) in the presence of submicronic inert carbon-black particles, they develop an acute pulmonary oedema and most of them die rapidly, usually in less than 6 hours.

This idea that the toxicity of sulphur mustard could be enhanced by the presence of particles was put forward again during the Iran–Iraq war, when chemical weapons were used on a large scale, and again in the Gulf War, when chemical weapons were not used. The concept is worth considering in some detail.

The toxicity of CW agents could be enhanced by absorption onto particles by the following mechanisms:

1. Sulphur mustard is absorbed mainly in the upper respiratory tract. The damage produced leads to incapacitation but is seldom fatal. The adsorption of sulphur mustard onto and slow release from small particles could lead to bypassing of the upper respiratory tract and the production of more serious damage in the gas-exchanging part of the lung.
2. Release of toxic materials from particles could lead to increased local concentrations of these substances and thus increased, though very localized, damage.
3. The duration of tissue exposure to toxic chemical might be increased by slow release from particles.

However, adsorption of toxic gases by particles without subsequent release would be expected to reduce toxicity. For substances which act systemically and do not produce their effect by damage to the lung, little is likely to be gained by adsorption onto particles. In addition, dilution of a toxic material with inert particles inevitably reduces the weapon payload of that toxic material.

Detailed experimental studies of the effects of adsorbing toxic materials onto particles have been undertaken, or at least reported, by only a very few workers. Probably the most detailed analysis reported is that of Goetz,[35] who worked largely from rather unsatisfactory data collected by LaBelle.[36] Goetz's analysis is considered below.

The surface area of a sphere is given by:

$$4\pi r^2 = \pi d^2$$

and its volume by:

$$\tfrac{4}{3}\pi r^3 = \tfrac{1}{6}\pi d^3 = 0.52 d^3$$

Let the mass of particles per unit volume of aerosol be C_p g l^{-1}, and let particle density be ρ. The mass of one particle is then:

$$\frac{\pi d^3 \rho}{6}$$

The number of particles per litre is given by:

$$\frac{6C_p}{\pi d^3 \rho}$$

The total surface area of particles, per litre of aerosol, is given by:

$$A_p = \frac{6C_p}{\pi d^3 \rho} \pi d^2$$

$$A_p = \frac{6C_p}{d\rho}$$

Let t = mean duration of survival of a group of animals exposed to toxic substance T in the absence of particles.

Let t_A = mean duration of survival of a group of animals exposed to toxic substance T in the presence of particles at a concentration of C_p g l^{-1}.

Let α', the relative synergistic effect of the aerosol, be defined as:

$$\alpha' = 1 - \frac{t_A}{t}$$

If α' is negative then the particles have an attenuating effect on the toxicity of T. If α' is positive then the particles have an intensifying effect upon the toxicity of T.

Let the specific effectiveness or synergistic potential of the particles be defined in terms of unit surface area by:

$$\alpha = \frac{\alpha'}{A_p}$$

$$\alpha = \frac{\alpha'}{A_p} = \frac{\rho d}{6 C_p} \left[1 - \frac{t_A}{t} \right]$$

This allows comparison of the effects of different particles upon the toxicity of substance T.

Data from LaBelle[36] with calculated values of α are shown for a range of toxic gases and a variety of particles in Table 21. In common with much of Goetz's paper,[35] the table and the associated calculations are difficult to follow. α seems to be expressed as a percentage. Values for A_p in the rows relating to nitric acid should be taken as the same as those shown for acrolein, and the original table contained a misprint: for acrolein and NaCl, $t_A = 71$ and not 0.71.

Goetz[35] summarized these findings in a shorter table (Table 22). It will be seen that the nature of the particle–toxicant interaction is dependent both upon the identity of the toxic material and that of the particles. Goetz reached the following conclusions:

1. In general the intensifying action of particles decreases with decreasing volatility of the toxic substance.
2. The porous particles, e.g. clay, act as intensifiers for very volatile materials such as formaldehyde but as attenuators for nitric acid.
3. Glycols and glycerol showed little effect.

Goetz[35] proceeded to develop a theoretical framework to explain the above observations. His argument is complex and the mathematical analysis, though rewarding, is bedevilled by a number of misprints. In essence his argument was that deposition of gas molecules from the gas phase on the respiratory surface would lead (unless gas concentrations were very high) to only a low percentage coverage of the surface, i.e. molecules would be widely spaced out on the surface. He argued that the irritant effect of the gas would be dependent upon the percentage areal coverage at any small part of the total respiratory surface. This might be disputed.

If, on the contrary, deposition of gas molecules occurred from the surface of a well-laden particle which had impacted upon the surface, then a much greater local areal coverage of the respiratory surface might be obtained. Goetz concluded from his model that synergism between toxicants and particles could occur but only in a comparatively narrow range of gas concentrations: he suggested that this was why the effect had not been more commonly observed in experimental work.[35]

It is a matter of regret that other authors have not followed up the work of Goetz. Recent experimental studies by Amdur[37] have shown that very fine metal-containing particles may enhance the effects of low concentrations of sulphur dioxide upon the guinea pig lung. Interestingly, the most sensitive index of effect was a change in the diffusing capacity of the guinea pig lung for carbon monoxide. This measure of lung function reflects the state of the diffusion barrier at the alveolar level and suggests that the sulphur dioxide, which is usually removed by the upper respiratory tract, penetrated to, and had effects upon, the distal lung. It would be interesting to know whether the combination of sulphur mustard with similar particles would have the same effect.

Table 21. Experimentally derived constants for calculation of synergistic potential

	Triethylene glycol	Ethylene glycol	Glycerol	Mineral oil	Silica gel	Clay	Dicalite	Celite	NaCl	Control
ρ (g cm^{-3})	1.1	1.1	1.3	0.8	1.4	2.5	2.1	2.1	2.1	
d (10^{-4} cm)	1.8	2.0	2.0	2.1	2.7	3.3	3.3	2.9	2.6	
Formaldehyde										
A_P (cm^2)	67	79	29.6	50	4.9	7.0	3.65	3.55	25.3	
t_A (min)	71	(168)	114	72	(145)	(157)	118	102	114	147
α	+0.775	(−0.177)	+0.78	+1.02	(+0.20)	(−0.71)	+5.5	+8.72	+0.91	—
Acrolein										
A_P (cm^2)	11.5	13.6	5.1	8.5	0.79	1.16	0.61	0.59	4.25	
t_A (min)	(73)	(106)	(94)	69	65	(78)	(91)	(99)	71	87
α	(+1.39)	(−1.62)	(−1.37)	+2.47	+31.7	(+0.86)	(−8.2)	−23.8	+4.22	—
Nitric acid										
t_A (min)	142	151	(103)	72	177	198	254	188	220	118
α	−1.74	−2.06	(+3.9)	+4.5	−63	−59	−189	−100	−20.2	—

Reprinted from *International Journal of Air and Water Pollution*, 4, A Goetz, On the nature of the synergistic action of aerosols, pp. 168–184, 1961, with kind permission from Elsevier Science Ltd, The Boulevard, Langford Lane, Kidlington OX5 1GB, UK
Data in parentheses are of no statistical significance.

Table 22. Synergistic potential of various aerosol types

	Formaldehyde	Acrolein	Nitric acid
Intensifying action	*Celite* Dicalite *Mineral oil* NaCl *Glycerol* *Triethylene glycol*	Silica gel NaCl Mineral oil	Mineral oil
Attenuating action	None	(Celite) (Dicalite)	*Dicalite* *Celite* *Silica gel* *Clay* *NaCl* *Ethylene glycol* *Triethylene glycol*

In italics: 'highly significant' data. In parentheses, data of no statistical significance if $\alpha > 5$.
Reprinted from *International Journal of Air and Water Pollution*, **4**, A Goetz, On the nature of the synergistic action of aerosols, pp. 168–184, 1961, with kind permission from Elsevier Science Ltd, The Boulevard, Langford Lane, Kidlington OX5 1GB, UK

REFERENCES

1. Comroe JH (1974) *Physiology of Respiration*, 2nd edn. Chicago: Year Book Medical Publishers.
2. Muir DCF (1972) *Clinical Aspects of Inhaled Particles*. London: William Heinemann Medical Books.
3. Green HL and Lane WR (1964) *Particulate Clouds: Dusts, Smokes and Mists*, 2nd edn. London: E. & H.F. Spon.
4. Starling SG (1935) *Mechanical Properties of Matter*. London: Macmillan and Co.
5. Florey H (1962) *General Pathology*, 3rd edn. London: Lloyd Luke (Medical Books).
6. Cocks AT and Fernando RP (1982) The growth of sulphate aerosols in the human airways. *J Aerosol Sci*, **13**, 9–19.
7. Pritchard JN (1987) Particle growth in the airways and the influence of airflow. In: *A New Concept in Inhalation Therapy* (SP Newman, F Morén and GK Crompton, eds), pp. 3–24. Proceedings of an international workshop on a new inhaler, 21–22 May 1987, London, UK. Bussum, London, München, Paris, Wien: Medicom.
8. Green H (1927) The effect of non-uniformity and particle shape on 'average particle size'. *J Franklin Inst*, **204**, 713–729.
9. Drinker P (1925) The size-frequency and identification of certain phagocytosed dusts. *J Ind Hyg*, **7**, 305.
10. Raabe OG (1970) Generation and characterization of aerosols. In: *Inhalation Carcinogenesis* (MG Hanna, P Nettershein and JR Gilbert, eds), pp. 123–172. Proceedings of a Biology Division, Oak Ridge National Laboratory Conference. Oak Ridge, Tennessee: US Atomic Energy Commission.
11. Hinds WC (1982) Particle size statistics. In: *Aerosol Technology. Properties, Behavior and Measurement of Airborne Particles*, pp. 69–103. New York, Chichester, Brisbane, Toronto, Singapore: John Wiley & Sons.
12. Hatch T and Choate SP (1929) Statistical description of the size properties of non-uniform particulate substances. *J Franklin Inst*, **207**, 369–387.

13. Hatch T (1933) Determination of 'average particle size' from the screen-analysis of non-uniform particulate substances. *J Franklin Inst*, **215**, 27–38.
14. Menzel DB and Amdur MO (1986) Toxic responses of the respiratory system. In: *Casarett and Doull's Toxicology: the Basic Science of Poisons*, 3rd edn (LJ Casarett, J Doull, CD Klaasen and MO Amdur, eds), pp. 330–358. London, New York: Macmillan.
15. Findeisen W (1935) Über das Absetzen kleiner in der Luft suspendierter Teilchen in der menschlichen Lunge bei der Atmung. *Pflüger's Arch Gesamte Physiol*, **236**, 367–379.
16. Stober W, McClellan RO and Morrow PE (1993) Approaches to modelling disposition of inhaled particles and fibres in the lung. In: *Toxicology of the Lung*, 2nd edn (DE Gardner, JD Crapo and RO McClellan, eds), pp. 527–602. New York: Raven Press.
17. Landahl HD (1950) On the removal of air-borne droplets by the human respiratory system. The lung. *Bull Math Biophys*, **12**, 43–56.
18. Hatch T and Hemeon WCL (1948) Influence of particle size in dust exposure. *J Ind Hyg Toxicol*, **30**, 172.
19. Altshuler B (1959) Calculation of regional deposition of aerosol in the respiratory tract. *Bull Math Biophys*, **21**, 257–270.
20. Task Group on Lung Dynamics (1966) Deposition and retention models for internal dosimetry of the human respiratory tract. *Health Phys*, **12**, 173–207.
21. Weibel ER (1963) *Morphometry of the Human Lung*. Berlin: Springer-Verlag.
22. Horsfield K and Cumming G (1967) Angles of branching and diameters of branches in the human bronchial tree. *Bull Math Biophys*, **29**, 245–259.
23. Horsfield K and Cumming C (1968) Morphology of the bronchial tree in man. *J Appl Physiol*, **24**, 373–383.
24. Valberg PA (1985) Determination of retained lung dose from toxicology of inhaled materials. In: *Handbook of Experimental Pharmacology*, Vol. 75 (H-P Witschi and JD Brain, eds), pp. 57–91. Berlin: Springer-Verlag.
25. Davies CN (ed.) (1966) *Aerosol Science*. New York: Academic Press.
26. Martonen TB, Barnett AE and Miller FJ (1985) Ambient sulfate aerosol deposition in man: modelling the influence of hygroscopicity. *Environ Health Perspect*, **63**, 11–24.
27. Kupprat I, Johnson R and Hertig B (1976) Ammonia: a normal constituent of expired air during rest and exercise. *Fed Proc Fed Am Soc Exp Biol*, **35**, 478.
28. Larson TV, Covert DS, Frank R et al. (1977) Ammonia in the human airways: neutralisation of inspired acid sulphate aerosols. *Science*, **197**, 161–163.
29. Cocks AT and McElroy WJ (1984) Modeling studies of the concurrent growth and neutralisation of sulfuric acid aerosols under conditions in the human airways. *Environ Res*, **35**, 79–96.
30. Muir DCF and Davies CN (1967) The deposition of 0.5 μ diameter aerosols in the lungs of man. *Ann Occup Hyg*, **10**, 161–174.
31. Dennis WL (1971) The effect of breathing rate on the deposition of particles in the human respiratory system. In: *Inhaled Particles, III* (WH Walton, ed.), pp. 91–102. Old Woking: Unwin.
32. Finney DJ (1952) *Probit Analysis: a Statistical Treatment of the Sigmoid Response Curve*, 2nd edn. Cambridge: Cambridge University Press.
33. Lefebure V (1921) *The Riddle of the Rhine*. London: W. Collins Sons & Co.
34. Dautrebande L (1962) *Microaerosols*. New York: Academic Press.
35. Goetz A (1961) On the nature of the synergistic action of aerosols. *Int J Air Water Poll*, **4**, 168–184.
36. LaBelle CW, Long JE and Christofano EE (1955) Synergistic effects of aerosols. Particulates as carriers of toxic vapours. *AMA Arch Ind Health*, **11**, 297–304.
37. Amdur MO, Chen LC, Guty J et al. (1988) Speciation and pulmonary effects of acidic SO_2 formed on the surface of ultrafine zinc with aerosols. *Atmos Environ*, **22**, 557–560.

3

ORGANOPHOSPHATE NERVE AGENTS

The organophosphate (OP) nerve agents are related to the OP pesticides, but have a much higher mammalian acute toxicity, particularly via the percutaneous route. Qualitatively the anticholinesterase toxicology of the OP nerve agents and pesticides is similar, and in general treatment strategies are alike.

HISTORY

OP compounds were intensively investigated in Germany in the 1930s. The German conglomerate IG Farbenindustrie looked at a number of these compounds for use as insecticides, and a program of synthesis of a large number of compounds was undertaken. Tabun and sarin, OPs of little use as insecticides but of very high mammalian toxicity, were synthesized by Schrader in 1937 and a small pilot production plant was set up at Münster-Lager. Subsequently, at Dühernfurt near Breslau in Prussian Silesia (now Dyhernfurth and Wrocław in Poland) a nerve agent production plant was built and both tabun and sarin were produced in quantity. Soman, another nerve agent, was also synthesized in Germany during the war, but only manufactured in small quantities. Strangely perhaps, in view of the large stocks held by Germany, the nerve agents were not used in World War II.[1] Other nerve agents were developed subsequently and stocks are held by a number of countries, including the USA, the former USSR, France and Iraq. However, nerve agents have rarely been used in warfare, the only notable instance of use being by Iraq against that country's own Kurdish population.[2] There have also been allegations of use of OP nerve agents during the Iran–Iraq war. The nerve agent sarin, almost certainly in an impure form, was used in two terrorist attacks in Japan, in Matsumoto and Tokyo in 1994 and 1995 respectively.

Possible roles of OP nerve agents are outlined in Table 1.

The nerve agents are traditionally divided into the G agents, GB (sarin, isopropyl methylphosphonofluoridate), GD (soman, pinacolyl methylphosphonofluoridate) and GA (tabun, ethyl, *N,N*-dimethylphosphoramidocyanidate), and the V agents, exemplified by VX (*O*-ethyl-*S*-[2-(diisopropylamino)ethyl] methylphosphonothio-

Table 1 Possible military targets for nerve agents

Target	Type of agent			Delivery system
	Sarin	Soman*	VX	
Rear area target				
Airports/Airfields		L	L	Aircraft: bombs, cluster spray bombs, spray tanks, missiles
Seaports		L	L	As above
Railway junctions		L	L	Aircraft: bombs, cluster
Headquarters and communication centers		L	L	Aircraft: bombs, missiles
Storage sites		L	L	Aircraft: bombs, cluster, missiles
Troop concentrations		L	L	Aircraft: bombs, spray tanks
Forward areas				
Nuclear delivery weapons, other key weapons and systems	L		L	Multiple rocket launchers, Aircraft: bombs, rockets
Defense positions	L		L	Multiple rocket launchers, artillery, mortars, aircraft bombs, rockets
Own flanks			L	Mines
Own defense front generally	L		L	Artillery, mortars, mines
To produce casualties, to harass and reduce combat efficiency	L		L	Multiple rocket launchers, artillery, mortars, aircraft: bombs, rockets
To deny unwanted ground		L	L	Aircraft: spray, mines
Harass civilian population	L			Aircraft: bombs, rockets, spray

* The Soman may be in a thickened form.
L = Likely use.
Adapted with permission from Maynard RL and Beswick F (1992) Organophosphorus compounds as chemical warfare agents. In: *Clinical and Experimental Toxicology of Organophosphates and Carbamates* (B Ballantyne and TC Marrs, eds), Butterworth Heinemann.

ate) (Table 2). These compounds differ amongst themselves in certain properties; for example, the V agents are less volatile than the G agents, a fact that may significantly affect their role in warfare. The toxic actions of all the nerve agents are very similar, although some differences have been observed. There are differences between the OPs with respect to their relative central and peripheral effects,[3,4] and, within the central nervous system (CNS), some differences between the OPs may exist. Thus Churchill *et al.*[5] noted significant dissimilarities in toxic responses and regional pattern of glucose utilization after soman and diisopropyl phosphorofluoridate (DFP) had been injected into rats. Differences also extend to treatment, where the inefficacy of oxime reactivators in soman poisoning and a similar lack of activity of pralidoxime in tabun poisoning are of great importance.

Plasma cholinesterase activity correlates badly with brain cholinesterase activity and is best thought of as a marker of poisoning rather than a prognostic indicator. Even activity of the preferred red cell acetylcholinesterase correlates poorly with central nervous acetylcholinesterase activity, seriously limiting the use of the former

Table 2 Formulae of nerve agents

Abbreviation	Common name	Proper name
GA	Tabun	Ethyl *N*-dimethylphosphoramidocyanidate

$$CH_3CH_2O\diagdown \overset{\displaystyle O}{\underset{\displaystyle \diagdown}{\overset{\parallel}{P}}}$$
$$(CH_3)_2N \diagup \quad \diagdown CN$$

| GB | Sarin | Isopropyl methylphosphonofluoridate |

$$\begin{array}{c} CH_3 \\ | \\ CH_3CHO \diagdown \quad \diagup O \\ P \\ CH_3 \diagup \quad \diagdown F \end{array}$$

| GD | Soman | Pinacolyl methylphosphonofluoridate |

$$\begin{array}{c} CH_3 \\ | \\ (CH_3)_3C-CHO \diagdown \quad \diagup O \\ P \\ CH_3 \diagup \quad \diagdown F \end{array}$$

| GE | — | Isopropyl ethylphosphonofluoridate |

$$\begin{array}{c} CH_3 \\ \diagdown \\ CHO \diagdown \quad \diagup O \\ CH_3 \diagup \qquad P \\ C_2H_5 \diagup \quad \diagdown F \end{array}$$

| GF | — | Cyclohexyl methylphosphonofluoridate |

$$\begin{array}{c} CH_2-CH_2 \\ \diagup \qquad \diagdown \\ CH_2 \qquad \qquad CHO \diagdown \quad \diagup O \\ \diagdown \qquad \diagup \qquad P \\ CH_2-CH_2 \qquad CH_3 \diagup \diagdown F \end{array}$$

| VX | — | *O*-Ethyl-*S*-[2(diisopropylamino)ethyl] methylphosphonothioate |

$$C_2H_5O\diagdown \quad \diagup O$$
$$P$$
$$CH_3 \diagup \quad \diagdown SCH_2CH_2N \underset{\diagdown CH(CH_3)_2}{\overset{\diagup CH(CH_3)_2}{}}$$

| VE | — | *O*-Ethyl-*S*-[2-(diethylamino)ethyl] ethylphosphonothioate |

$$C_2H_5O\diagdown \quad \diagup O$$
$$P$$
$$C_2H_5 \diagup \quad \diagdown SCH_2CH_2N(C_2H_5)_2$$

(*continued overleaf*)

Table 2 (*continued*)

Abbreviation	Common name	Proper name
VG	—	*O,O*-Diethyl-*S*-[2-(diethylamino)ethyl] phosphorothioate
VM	—	*O*-Ethyl-*S*-[2-(diethylamino)ethyl] methylphosphonothioate

For VG:

$$C_2H_5O \diagdown \underset{C_2H_5O}{\overset{\displaystyle \nearrow O}{P}} \diagdown SCH_2CH_2N(C_2H_5)_2$$

For VM:

$$C_2H_5O \diagdown \underset{CH_3}{\overset{\displaystyle \nearrow O}{P}} \diagdown SCH_2CH_2N(C_2H_5)_2$$

Adapted with permission from Maynard RL and Beswick F (1992) Organophosphorus compounds as chemical warfare agents. In: *Clinical and Experimental Toxicology of Organophosphates and Carbamates* (B Ballantyne and TC Marrs, eds), Butterworth-Heinemann.

to assess the severity of poisoning.[6] With nerve agents, for example soman, there is some indication that there are differences in the sensitivities of different acetylcholinesterases within the nervous system.[7]

CHEMISTRY AND PHYSICAL PROPERTIES

The nerve agents comprise a group of OPs of high acute mammalian toxicity. They are derivatives of phosphoric or phosphonic acids and contain two alkyl groups and a leaving group. In the case of the G agents the leaving group is often a fluorine atom and, exceptionally in GE, one of the alkyl groups is replaced by a cyclohexyl group. Soman is distinguished by the fact that one of its alkyl groups is a bulky pinocolyl group, while tabun does not contain a fluorine atom and its leaving group is a CN moiety. Tabun is notably easier to synthesize in bulk than sarin and soman. Incorporation of the fluorine leaving group requires the use of hydrofluoric acid during the synthesis and this is, of course, corrosive to glass. Early bulk synthesis of nerve agents with fluorine leaving groups was carried out using special apparatus made or lined with pure silver. Such a process is inevitably costly. It is of interest that the nerve agent likely to have been used by Iraq against Kurds was tabun: the first nerve agent to be synthesized on a large scale (Chapter 1). The V agents are phosphonothioates of the P=O type in which the leaving group is linked to phosphorus through a sulfur atom, except for VG which is a phosphorothioate. The formulae of the G and V agents are given in Table 2. All are colorless liquids, although impure agents may be yellow to brown. The G agents are volatile liquids (tabun less volatile than sarin or soman), whilst VX is a non-volatile liquid (Table 3). Tabun is said to have a fruity odor, while the other agents are said to be odorless.

Table 3 Physicochemical properties of nerve agents

		Tabun GA		Sarin GB		Soman GD		VX		GF	
Molecular weight		162.3		140.1		182.18		267.36		180.14	
Specific gravity at 25°C		1.073		1.0087		1.022		1.0083		1.133[1]	
Boiling point (°C)		246		147		167		300		—	
Melting point (°C)		−49		−56		−80		−20		−12	
Vapour pressure (VP) and volatility (Vol)	°C	VP (mmHg)	Vol (mg m^{-3})	VP (mmHg)	Vol (mg m^{-3})	VP (mmHg)	Vol (mg m^{-3})	VP (mmHg)	Vol (mg m^{-3})	VP (mmHg)	Vol (mg m^{-3})
	0	0.004	38	0.52	4 279.0	0.044	470.9			0.006	63
	10	0.013	119.5	1.07	8 494.0	0.11	1135.5			0.017	173
	20	0.036	319.8	2.10	16 101.0	0.27	2692.1	0.00044	5.85†	0.044	434
	25	0.07	611.3	2.9	21 862.0	0.40	3921.4	0.0007	10.07	0.068	659
	30	0.094	807.4	3.93	29 138.0	0.61	5881.4			0.104	991
	40	0.23	1912.4	7.1	60 959.0	—	—			0.234	2159
	50	0.56	4512.0	12.3	83 548.0	2.60	23516.0			0.501	4480

[1] temp = 20°C.

Volatility = concentration of saturated vapor at specified temperature. Volatility calculated from $PV = nRT$ (see Chapter 2).

$$Vol = \frac{VP \times 101\,325 \times MW}{760 \times 8.3143 \times A} = \frac{VP \times MW \times 16.035}{A}$$

A = absolute temperature.

† Some authorities quote values as low as 0.1–1.0 mg m^{-3}.

Adapted with permission from Maynard RL and Beswick F (1992) Organophosphorus compounds as chemical warfare agents. In: *Clinical and Experimental Toxicology of Organophosphates and Carbamates* (B Ballantyne and TC Marrs, eds), Butterworth-Heinemann.

TOXICOLOGY

Acute

Acute toxicity figures are available for nerve agents in many species (Table 4). The acute toxic dose in humans is not known with any exactitude, as poisoning with nerve agents has only rarely been observed in humans.[11,39] Therefore lethal doses and likely clinical effects in humans have to be inferred from experimental poisoning in animals and from OP pesticide poisoning. The cases that have been studied, together with low-dose volunteer studies with nerve agents, do not suggest any major differences between humans and other animals in clinical response to nerve agents.

Toxicological actions

The action of OP nerve agents on the nervous system results from their effects on enzymes, particularly esterases. The most notable of these esterases is acetylcholinesterase, where the OPs phosphorylate a serine hydroxyl group in the active site of the enzyme. The normal function of acetylcholinesterase is to destroy acetylcholine in the synaptic cleft or neuromuscular junction, in order to terminate transmission of a nerve impulse: failure of acetylcholinesterase activity results in accumulation of acetylcholine,[40,41] which in turn causes enhancement and prolongation of cholinergic effects and also depolarization blockade. Reactivation of acetylcholinesterase occurs by dephosphorylation, and the rates of phosphorylation and dephosphorylation are very variable, which partly accounts for differences in acute toxicity between the nerve agents. The hydrolysis reaction for acetylated acetylcholinesterase is fast: the half-life of the acetylated enzyme was given by Koelle as 42 μs. Hydrolysis of acetylcholinesterases carbamylated by carbamates such as neostigmine, physostigmine and pyridostigmine proceeds much more slowly: Koelle gave 30 min as the half-life of the enzyme–neostigmine complex. With some organophosphorylated acetylcholinesterases (but notably not OP insecticides), hydrolysis is even slower: DFP-inhibited enzyme hydrolyzes extremely slowly, so slowly in fact that the binding of the organophosphate to the enzyme has been described as irreversible. This is an inappropriate term. With soman, the situation is further complicated by an additional reaction known as aging. This consists of monodealkylation of the dialkylphosphonyl enzyme, creating a much more stable monoalkylphosphonyl enzyme, the reactivation rate of which is negligible. Soman produces an inhibited acetylcholinesterase which ages very rapidly by loss of the large pinacolyl group, with the result that reactivation of inhibited acetylcholinesterase does not occur to any clinically significant extent. Therefore, in the case of soman, recovery of function depends on resynthesis of acetylcholinesterase.[42] With other OPs where aging occurs more slowly, reactivation is relatively rapid; however, where treatment is instituted late, or where there has been repeated exposure, significant amounts of enzyme may be in the aged state. The slow aging process which occurs in regard to tabun and sarin has been taken by some to indicate that treatment can be safely delayed. Nothing could be further from the truth. Aging has little to do with the toxic effects

Table 4 Comparative acute toxicity of nerve agents

Species	Route	Term	Unit	Tabun	Sarin	Soman	VX
Man	PC	LD_{50}	mg kg^{-1}		28[8]		
	PC	LCLO	μg kg^{-1}				86[9]
	PC	LDLO	mg kg^{-1}	23[8]		18[8]	
	inhal	LDLO	mg m^{-3}	150[8]		70[8]	
	inhal	LD_{50}	mg m^{-3}		70[8]		
	inhal	LDLO	μg m^{-3}		90[10]		
	IV	TDLO	μg kg^{-1}	14[8]			
	IV	TDLO	μg kg^{-1}				1.5[11]
	oral	TDLO	μg kg^{-1}		2[12]		4[11]
	SC	LDLO	μg kg^{-1}				30[13]
	IM	TDLO	μg kg^{-1}				3.2[13]
Rat	PC	LD_{50}	mg kg^{-1}	18[14]			
	inhal	LC_{50}	mg m^{-3}/10 min	304[14]	150[10]		
	IV	LD_{50}	μg kg^{-1}	66[14]	39[15]	44.5[16]	
	oral	LD_{50}	μg kg^{-1}	3700[14]	550[14]		12[19]
	SC	LD_{50}	μg kg^{-1}	193[16]	103[17]	75[18]	
	IM	LD_{50}	μg kg^{-1}	800[12]	108[20]	62[20]	
	IP	LD_{50}	μg kg^{-1}		218[15]	98[21]	
Mouse	PC	LD_{50}	mg kg^{-1}	1[14]	1.08[14]		
	inhal	LC_{50}	mg m^{-3}/30 min	15[14]	5[22]	1[22]	
	IV	LD_{50}	μg kg^{-1}	150[14]	113[23]	35[24]	
	SC	LD_{50}	μg kg^{-1}	250[25]	60[22]	40[22]	22[25]
	SC	LD_{50}	μg kg^{-1}		172[37]		
	IM	LD_{50}	μg kg^{-1}	440[23]	222[23]		
	IP	LD_{50}	μg kg^{-1}		420[27]	393[27]	50[9]
Dog	PC	LD_{50}	mg kg^{-1}	30[14]			
	inhal	LC_{50}	mg m^{-3}/10 min	400[14]	100[14]		
	IV	LD_{50}	μg kg^{-1}	84[28]	19[28]		
	oral	LD_{50}	μg kg^{-1}	200[22]			
	SC	LD_{50}	μg kg^{-1}	284[18]		12[29]	
Monkey	PC	LD_{50}	μg kg^{-1}	9300[14]			
	inhal	LC_{50}	mg m^{-3}/10 min	250[14]	100[14]		
	SC	LD_{50}	μg kg^{-1}			13[30]	
	IM	LD_{50}	μg kg^{-1}		22.3[31]	9.5[32]	
Cat	inhal	LC_{50}	mg m^{-3}/10 min	250[14]	100[28]		
	IV	LD_{50}	μg kg^{-1}		22[14]		
Rabbit	PC	LD_5	μg kg^{-1}	2500[14]	925[14]		
	inhal	LC_{50}	mg m^{-3}/10 min	840[14]	120[14]		
	IV	LD_{50}	μg kg^{-1}	63[14]	15[33]		
	oral	LD_{50}	μg kg^{-1}	16300[14]			
	SC	LD_{50}	μg kg^{-1}	375[34]	30[35]	20[29]	14[36]
	IP	LD_{50}	μg kg^{-1}				66[36]

(*continued overleaf*)

Table 4 (*continued*)

Species	Route	Term	Unit	Tabun	Sarin	Soman	VX
Guinea pig	PC	LD_{50}	mg kg^{-1}	35[14]			
	inhal	LC_{50}	mg m^{-3}/2 min	393[14]			
	SC	LD_{50}	mg kg^{-1}	120[35]			
	SC	LD_{50}	μg kg^{-1}		30[34]	24[35]	8.4[35]
Hamster	SC	LD_{50}	μg kg^{-1}	245[38]	95[34]		
Farm	PC	LD_{50}	μg kg^{-1}	1100[14]			
animal	inhal	LC_{50}	mg m^{-3}/14 min	400[14]			
Chickens	SC	LD_{50}	μg kg^{-1}			50[21]	
	IP	LD_{50}	μg kg^{-1}			71[29]	
Frog	IP	LD_{50}	μg kg^{-1}			251[21]	

PC, percutaneous; inhal, inhalation; IV, intravenous; SC, subcutaneous; IM, intramuscular; IP, intraperitoneal.
Adapted with permission from Maynard RL and Beswick F (1992) Organophosphorus compounds as chemical warfare agents. In: *Clinical and Experimental Toxicology of Organophosphates and Carbamates* (B Ballantyne and TC Marrs, eds), Butterworth-Heinemann.

of OPs: these are of course dependent on the accumulation of acetylcholine at essential sites.

The clinical effects of nerve agents are, to a large extent, those of acetylcholine accumulation, and the effects of all the nerve agents are similar. Those differences that have been observed are presumably due to a combination of different rates of inactivation and reactivation of the enzymes, together with different rates of aging of the inhibited enzyme and differences in pharmacokinetics, distribution and metabolism of the nerve agent. It is noteworthy that in the case of soman, kinetic differences have been recorded between the different stereoisomers.[43]

The symptoms and signs of nerve agent poisoning may be divided into three groups, muscarinic (postganglionic parasympathetic receptors), nicotinic (preganglionic sympathetic and parasympathetic terminals and the neuromuscular junction) and central (Table 5). The muscarinic symptoms and signs result from increased activity of the parasympathetic system and include bronchorrhea, salivation, constriction of the pupil of the eye (miosis), abdominal colic and bradycardia.[44] Nicotinic effects at autonomic ganglia can produce pallor, tachycardia and hypertension. The clinical effects in the cardiovascular system depend on whether muscarinic or nicotinic effects predominate. At the neuromuscular junction, nicotinic signs include muscle fasciculation and later paralysis. If the patient survives the acute cholinergic syndrome, the effects of nerve agents are largely reversible, although, as discussed above, with soman recovery may be very slow and in certain circumstances there may be long-term changes in the CNS (see below).

Miosis is the term used to describe the constriction of the pupil. The term is often assumed to be derived from the same Greek root as meiosis, i.e. a diminution. This is in fact not the case. Miosis, and the earlier variant myosis, are derived from the Greek root myein (or muein): to close, blink (Shorter Oxford English Dictionary, Webster's Third New International Dictionary).

Table 5 Main effects of nerve agents at various sites in the body

Receptor	Target organ	Symptoms and signs
Central	Central nervous system	Giddiness, anxiety, restlessness, headache, tremor, confusion, failure to concentrate, convulsions, respiratory depression
Muscarinic	Glands	
	Nasal mucosa	Rhinorrhea
	Bronchial mucosa	Bronchorrhea
	Sweat	Sweating
	Lacrimal	Lacrimation
	Salivary	Salivation
	Smooth Muscle	
	Iris	Miosis
	Ciliary muscle	Failure of accommodation
	Gut	Abdominal cramp, diarrhea
	Bladder	Frequency, involuntary micturition
	Heart	Bradycardia
Nicotinic	Autonomic ganglia	Sympathetic effects, pallor, tachycardia, hypertension
	Skeletal muscle	Weakness, fasciculation

Where death occurs, it is caused by respiratory paralysis, which may be central or due to the anticholinesterase action at the neuromuscular junction.[45]

NON-ANTICHOLINESTERASE EFFECTS

Clinically, the most important effects of OP nerve agents are anticholinesterase actions. However, there is some evidence that some OPs can act directly on muscarinic receptors.[46,47] It has also been demonstrated that OPs, including nerve agents, can affect pathways other than cholinergic ones, for example dopaminergic and somatostatinergic.[48–52] It is possible that some of the CNS effects of nerve agents are secondary to changes in the blood–brain barrier.

Effects on specific organs

THE EYE

Nerve agents produce miosis; this produces a feeling that the surroundings are dim, or that illumination has been reduced. The onset is rapid and may last for several days. Spasm of the ciliary muscle may impair accommodation. Long-lasting miosis, associated with eye pain, was a notable clinical sign in the Tokyo subway (underground railway) terrorist attack with sarin.

Dilatation of subconjunctival blood vessels occurs and the eye becomes bloodshot. After exposure to high concentrations of nerve agent the eyes take on a glassy appearance: the appearance is sometimes compared to that of a glass marble. The lacrimal glands do not seem to be much affected by exposure to nerve agent vapor and tearing is not a reliable early sign of exposure.

THE RESPIRATORY TRACT

The upper respiratory tract contains two components that are under cholinergic control. These are the mucous glands and smooth muscle. The response to nerve agents by the former is to increase secretions, resulting in bronchorrhea and rhinorrhea (runny nose). The effect on smooth muscle is to produce bronchospasm.

PERIPHERAL NERVOUS SYSTEM AND SKELETAL MUSCLE

Systemically, nerve agents produce fasciculation and then blockade at the neuromuscular junction, with weakness and paralysis. Some of these effects may be mediated by direct actions at the receptor–ion channel complex.

Separate from the acute effects of anticholinesterases upon the neuromuscular junction, two further syndromes involving the neuromuscular system have been associated with OP poisoning. These are (1) the intermediate syndrome and (2) OP-induced delayed neuropathy (OPIDN).

Intermediate syndrome

Senanayake and Karalliedde[53] described a new form of neurotoxicity following intoxication by organophosphorus insecticides. As it occurred after the acute syndrome and before the onset of classical OPIDN, they called it the 'intermediate syndrome'. This phenomenon consists of marked weakness of the proximal skeletal musculature (including the muscles of respiration) and cranial nerve palsies; it comes on 1–4 days after acute poisoning. Respiratory support is often necessary and, if it is provided, recovery occurs within 4–18 days. Although the intermediate syndrome has not been described in cases of accidental nerve agent poisoning, it is likely that it would occur at least in some cases. Intermediate syndrome is probably a consequence of cholinergic overactivity at the neuromuscular junction and a connection has been made between the intermediate syndrome and OP-induced myopathy.[54] Myopathy associated with OPs was first observed many years ago[55] and has been observed histologically in experimental animals with the nerve agents tabun and soman[56–58] and sarin.[37,59] The changes characteristic of OP-induced delayed neuropathy seem to be initiated by calcium influx[60] as a consequence of acetylcholine accumulation at the neuromuscular junction.[61,62] If it is these histological changes that underlie the intermediate syndrome, the development of the syndrome can be anticipated in the recovery phase of nerve agent poisoning in at least some cases.

Nerve-agent-induced delayed neuropathy

OP-induced delayed neuropathy (OPIDN) is a symmetrical sensorimotor axonopathy, tending to be most severe in long axons and occurring 7–14 days after exposure to OPs. In severe cases it is an extremely disabling condition. Inhibition of neuropathy target esterase (NTE), an esterase of unknown function present at several sites, including neurons, appears to be necessary for OPIDN to develop. This is followed by an aging reaction similar to that described for soman with acetylcholinesterase above.[63] By contrast with intermediate syndrome, it is extremely unlikely that nerve agents possess the capability to cause OPIDN. In experimental studies nerve agents do not bring about OPIDN.[64–67] The probable reason why nerve agents are non-neuropathic is that concentrations of nerve agent required to produce acetylcholinesterase inhibition are low, while those required for inhibition of NTE are relatively high, the reverse of the case with the neuropathic OPs such as mipafox, tri-*O*-cresyl phosphate or DFP.[68] Furthermore, in the case of soman, Johnson *et al.*[65] have shown that only a tiny proportion of inhibited NTE from hen brain and spinal cord undergoes aging. Moreover, structure–activity considerations lend no support to suggestions that nerve agents would be neuropathic.[69]

HEART

The acute effect on the heart depends on the relative predominance of muscarinic or nicotinic effects. Bradycardia or tachycardia may occur, as well as arrhythmias, including atrioventricular block and various ventricular arrhythmias. An arrhythmia characteristic of OP poisoning with pesticides is torsade de pointes,[70] while soman and other OPs have been reported to produce histopathological changes in the myocardium.[71,72]

CENTRAL NERVOUS SYSTEM

The nerve agents produce a wide range of effects upon the CNS, ranging from anxiety and emotional lability at low doses to convulsions and respiratory paralysis at higher ones. It is important to note that doses considerably below the LD_{50} can markedly degrade performance of tasks in behavioral studies,[31,73,74] and there is evidence that the decremental effects of exposure to single doses of nerve agents may be prolonged.[75] Clearly this is of importance, as it is likely that the military performance of personnel would be impaired: affected servicemen might not only lose the motivation to fight but also lose the ability to defend themselves and be unable to carry out the complex tasks frequently required in the modern armed forces. Effects on skilled personnel such as pilots and navigators would be particularly disabling.

The changes induced by nerve agents in the CNS are theoretically reversible and histopathological changes are few. Thus Anzueto *et al.*[76] found that, in baboons given intravenous infusions of soman, only minimal CNS pathology was observed. Not only does this absence of specific changes make diagnosis at autopsy difficult, but it also implies that complete recovery after successful treatment is to be expected. However, where humans survive high but sublethal doses of nerve agents it is probable that both histopathological changes and functional deficits would be observed. In animals, after soman the initial changes seen are edema, particularly astrocytic and perivascular hemorrhages. Neuronal degeneration and necrosis, sometimes diffuse, may be observed, together with more discrete infarcts, with necrosis of all cell types. Such changes may be detected particularly in the hippocampus and piriform cortex.[77] This picture, which does not seem to correlate with areas in which the blood–brain barrier is compromised, may proceed to an encephalopathy. Most commonly this affects the cortex, hippocampus and thalamic nuclei, a distribution that suggests anoxia is a likely cause.[71,75,77] The hypothesis that hypoxia secondary to convulsions is the cause is supported by the fact that the effects have been correlated with seizure activity[76] and that the anticonvulsant diazepam alleviates the effects.[78] Nevertheless, some authorities have disagreed with the attribution of nerve-agent-induced pathological changes to hypoxia and/or convulsions.[79] In view of these findings it is unsurprising that severe nerve agent poisoning is sometimes associated with long-term CNS changes both in experimental animals and in humans.[80-84] More debatable is whether lower doses, particularly subconvulsive ones, can bring about long-term changes in CNS function. A number of studies have been performed to investigate subtle changes in humans exposed to various sorts of OPs.[75,85-90] Many of these studies refer to OP insecticides, but those involving nerve agents are summarized in Table 6. A notable study involving nerve agents was carried out by Duffy et al.[91] Behavioral signs and subtle EEG changes were noted after exposure to sarin, severe enough to cause symptoms and clinical signs. Burchfiel et al.[92] described changes, which persisted for a year, in the EEGs of rhesus monkeys after a single large dose or repeated small doses of sarin. The lower dose used was 1 μg given by 10 weekly injections (total dose 10 μg = 7% LD$_{50}$). This result, which is somewhat surprising, must be interpreted cautiously as the group size was small (three per group) and similar but not identical EEG changes were seen after the organochlorine pesticide dieldrin, namely a relative increase in beta activity.

There seems very little doubt, on theoretical, experimental and epidemiological grounds, that severe OP poisoning can cause long-term irreversible changes in brain

Table 6 Summary of published work on long-term effects of nerve agents

	Exposed	Result	Controls	OP
Duffy et al.[91]	Workers	+ ve (EEG, multivariate analysis)	Non-exposed	Sarin
Burchfiel et al.[92]	Primates	+ ve EEG	Control animal + pre-exposure EEG	Sarin
Holmes and Gaon[80]	Workers	EEG changes	None Anecdote	OPI* Sarin DFP
McDonough et al.[75]	Rats	Behavioral decrement	Control animals	Soman

* OPI = mixed OP insecticides.

function. In less severe poisoning the data are conflicting: while there is some evidence of persistent EEG effects, in particular increased beta activity, few of the relevant studies are above criticism. The most impressive studies relate to sarin, but even here there is room for doubt and further work upon the subject is required. The implications for treatment are, at this time, uncertain; the most logical course would be to avoid anoxia as much as possible during treatment.

Effect of route of exposure

VAPOR

Onset is rapid and the eyes and respiratory system are most affected. Low-level exposure causes tightness of the chest, rhinorrhea and salivation. Dimming of vision due to miosis, eye pain and headache then follow. On examination the pupils are constricted and the conjunctivae hyperemic. These effects may last several hours after cessation of exposure and the headache and visual problems several days. In severe cases salivation and rhinorrhea are more marked, and wheezing and dyspnea are prominent. Other effects such as abdominal pain, vomiting, involuntary defecation and micturition, weakness, fasciculation and convulsion follow, depending on the degree of systemic absorption. Death may occur from respiratory failure.

The attack with sarin on the Tokyo subway (underground railway) has added considerably to our knowledge of the clinical effects of sarin vapor. The symptoms observed were largely as expected: cough, difficulty in breathing and tightness of the chest, bradycardia and eye pain.[93,94]

SKIN CONTAMINATION

Local effects at the site of contamination include sweating and local fasciculation. Fasciculation may spread to involve whole muscle groups, while the onset of systemic symptoms and signs is slower than after vapor exposure.

INGESTION

Ingestion of nerve agent may occur from contaminated food or water. Colicky pain occurs, together with nausea, vomiting, diarrhea and involuntary defecation.

CONCLUSION

The organophosphate nerve agents continue to pose major problems in chemical defense. Important measures in prevention of casualties include adequate detection measures, physical protection, chemical prophylaxis and proper treatment. Treatment of poisoning by organophosphorus nerve agents is dealt with in Chapter 4.

REFERENCES

1. UK Ministry of Defence (1972) *Medical Manual of Defence against Chemical Agents* JSP 312 A/24/Gen/4392, pp. 7–12. London, Edinburgh and Belfast: Her Majesty's Stationery Office.
2. le Chêne E (1989) Chemical and biological warfare—threat of the future. Mackenzie Paper. Toronto, Canada: The Mackenzie Institute.
3. Ligtenstein DA (1984) On the synergism of the cholinesterase reactivating bispyridinium-aldoxime HI-6 and atropine in the treatment of organophosphate intoxications in the rat. MD Thesis, University of Leyden, The Netherlands.
4. Misulis KE, Clinton ME, Dettbarn W-D and Gupta RC (1987) Differences in central and peripheral neural actions between soman and diisopropyl fluorophosphate, organophosphorus inhibitors of acetylcholinesterases. *Toxicol Appl Pharmacol*, **89**, 391–398.
5. Churchill L, Pazdernik TL, Cross RS *et al.* (1987) Cholinergic systems influence local cerebral glucose use in specific anatomical areas: diisopropyl phosphorofluoridate versus soman. *Neuroscience*, **20**, 329–339.
6. Jimmerson VR, Shih T-M and Mailman RB (1989) Variability in soman toxicity in the rat: correlation with biochemical and behavioral measures. *Toxicology*, **57**, 241–254.
7. Sellström Å, Algers G and Karlsson B (1985) Soman intoxication and the blood–brain barrier. *Fund Appl Toxicol*, **5**, S122–S126.
8. Robinson JP (1967) Chemical warfare. *Sci J*, **3**, 33–40.
9. WHO (1970) Technical Report. Health Aspects of Chemicals and Biological Weapons: report of a World Health Organization Group of Consultants. Geneva: World Health Organization.
10. Rengstorff HH (1985) Accidental exposure to sarin: vision effects. *Arch Toxicol*, **56**, 201–203.
11. Sidell FR (1974) Soman and sarin: clinical manifestations and treatment of accidental poisoning. *Clin Toxicol*, **7**, 1–17.
12. Grob D and Harvey AM (1958) Effects in man of the anticholinesterase compound sarin (isopropyl methyl phosphonofluoridate). *J Clin Invest*, **37**, 350–368.
13. National Academy of Sciences (1982) *Possible Long-term Health Effects of Short-term Exposure to Chemical Agents*, Vol. 1, *Anticholinesterases and Anticholinergics*, pp. 1–6. Washington DC: National Academy of Sciences.
14. Gates M and Renshaw BC (1946) Fluorophosphates and other phosphorus-containing compounds. In: *Summary Technical Report of Division 9*, Vol. 1, Parts I, II, pp. 131, 155. Washington DC: Office of Scientific Research & Development.
15. Fleisher J (1963) Effects of p-nitrophenyl phosphonate (EPN) on the toxicity of isopropyl methyl phosphonofluoridate (GB). *J Pharmacol Exp Ther*, **139**, 390.
16. Padzernik TL, Cross R, Nelson S *et al.* (1983) Soman-induced depression of brain activity in TAB-pretreated rats: 2-dooxyglucose study. *Neurotoxicity*, **4**, 27–34.
17. Brimblecombe RW, Green DM, Stratton JA and Thompson PB (1970) The protective actions of some anticholinergic drugs in sarin poisoning. *Br J Pharmacol*, **39**, 822–830.
18. Bosković B, Kovacević V and Jovanović D (1984) 2-PAM chloride, H16 and HGG 12 in soman and tabun poisoning. *Fund Appl. Toxicol*, **4**, 106–115.
19. Jovanović D (1982) The effect of bis-pyridinium oximes on neuromuscular blockade induced by highly toxic organophosphates in the rat. *Arch Int Pharmacodyn Ther*, **262**, 231–241.

20. Schoene K, Hochrainer D, Oldiges H *et al.* (1985) The protective effect of oxime pretreatment upon the inhalative toxicity of sarin and soman in rats. *Fund Appl Toxicol*, **5**, 584–588.

21. Chatthopadhay DP, Dighe SK, Nashikkar AB and Dube DK (1986) Species differences in the *in vitro* inhibition of brain acetylcholinesterase and carboxyl esterase by mipafox, paraoxon and soman. *Pestic Biochem Physiol*, **26**, 202–208.

22. Lotts von K (1960) Zur Toxikologie und pharmakologie organischer Phosphosäurester. *Dtsch Gesundheitsweren*, **15**, 2133–2179.

23. Schoene K and Oldiges H (1973) Efficacy of pyridinium salts against tabun and sarin poisoning *in vivo* and *in vitro*. *Arch Int Pharmacol Ther*, **204**, 110–123.

24. Brezenoff HE, McGee J and Knight V (1984) The hypertensive response to soman and its relation to brain acetylcholinesterase inhibition. *Acta Pharmacol Toxicol*, **55**, 270–277.

25. Maksimović M, Bosković B, Rodović L *et al.* (1980) Antidotal effects of bis pyridinium 2 mono oxime carbonyl derivatives in intoxication with highly toxic organophosphorus compounds. *Acute Pharm Jagoslav*, **30**, 151–160.

26. Fredriksson T (1957) Pharmacological properties of methyl fluorophosphonylcholines, two synthetic cholinergic drugs. *Arch Int Pharmacodyn Ther*, **113**, 101–104.

27. Clement JG (1984) Role of antiesterase in organophosphate poisoning. *Fund Appl Toxicol*, **4**, S96–S105.

28. O'Leary TF, Kunkel AM and Jones AH (1961) Efficacy and limitations of oxime–atropine treatment of organophosphorus anticholinesterase poisoning. *J Pharmacol Exp Ther*, **132**, 50–52.

29. Berry WK and Davies DR (1970) Use of carbamates and atropine in the protection of animals against poisoning by 1,2,2-trimethylpropyl phosphonofluoridate. *Biochem Pharmacol*, **19**, 927–934.

30. Clement JG, Hand BT and Shiloff JD (1981) Differences in the toxicity of soman in various strains of mice. *Fund Appl Toxicol*, **1**, 419–420.

31. D'Mello GD and Duffy EAM (1985) The acute toxicity of sarin in marmosets (*Callithrix jacchus*): a behavioral analysis. *Fund Appl Toxicol*, **5**, S169–S174.

32. Lipp SA (1972) Effect of diazepam upon soman induced seizure activities and convulsions. *Electroenceph Clin Neurophysiol*, **32**, 557–560.

33. Wills JH (1961) Anticholinergic compounds as adjuncts to atropine in preventing lethality by sarin in the rabbit. *J Med Pharmacol Chem*, **3**, 353–359.

34. Coleman IW, Patton GE and Bannard RA (1968) Cholinolytics in the treatment of anticholinesterase poisoning V. The effectiveness of parpanit with oximes in the treatment of organophosphorus poisoning. *Can J Physiol Pharmacol*, **46**, 109–117.

35. Gordon JJ and Leadbeater LL (1977) The prophylactic use of (1-methyl 2-hydroxyiminomethylpyridinium methanesulfonate) (P2S) in the treatment of organophosphate poisoning. *Toxicol Appl Pharmacol*, **40**, 109–114.

36. Leblic C, Cox HM and le Moan L (1984) Etude de la toxicité, de l'eserine, VX et le paraoxon, pour établir un modèle mathematique de l'extrapolation àtre humain. *Arch Blg Med Soc Hyg Trav Med Suppl*, 226–242.

37. Bright JE, Inns RH, Tuckwell NJ *et al.* (1991) A histochemical study of changes observed in the mouse diaphragm after organophosphate poisoning. *Human Exp Toxicol*, **10**, 9–14.

38. Coleman IW, Little PE, Patton GE and Bannard RHB (1966) Cholinolytics in the treatment of anticholinesterase poisoning IV. The effectiveness of five binary combinations of cholinolytics with oximes in the treatment of organophosphorus poisoning. *Can J Physiol*, **44**, 743–764.

39. Maynard RL and Beswick FW (1992) Organophosphorus compounds as chemical warfare agents. In: *Clinical and Experimental Toxicology of Organophosphates and*

Carbamates (B Ballantyne and TC Marrs, eds), pp. 373–385. Oxford: Butterworth-Heinemann.

40. Burgen ASV and Hobbiger F (1951) The inhibition of cholinesterases by alkylphosphates and alkylphenophosphates. *Br J Pharmacol Chemother*, **6**, 593–605.

41. Koelle GB (1992) Pharmacology and toxicology of organophosphates. In: *Clinical and Experimental Toxicology of Organophosphates and Carbamates* (B Ballantyne and TC Marrs, eds), pp. 33–37. Oxford: Butterworth-Heinemann.

42. Gray AP (1984) Design and structure–activity relationships of antidotes to organophosphorus anticholinesterase agents. *Drug Metab Rev*, **15**, 557–589.

43. Benschop HP, Bijleveld EC, de Jong LPA *et al.* (1987) Toxicokinetics of the four stereoisomers of the nerve agent soman in atropinized rats—influence of a soman simulator. *Toxicol Appl Pharmacol*, **90**, 490–500.

44. Grob D and Harvey AM (1953) The effects and treatment of nerve gas poisoning. *Am J Med*, **14**, 52–63.

45. Chang F-CT, Foster RE, Beers ET *et al.* (1990) Neurophysiological concomitants of soman-induced respiratory depression in awake, behaving guinea pigs. *Toxicol Appl Pharmacol*, **102**, 233–250.

46. Silveira CLP, Eldefrawi AT and Eldefrawi ME (1990) Putative M2 muscarinic receptors of rat heart have high affinity for organophosphorus anticholinesterases. *Toxicol Appl Pharmacol*, **103**, 474–481.

47. Mobley PL (1990) The cholinesterase inhibitor soman increases inositol triphosphate in rat brain. *Neuropharmacology*, **29**, 189–191.

48. Lau W-M, Freeman SE and Szilagyí M (1988) Binding of some organophosphorus compounds at adenosine receptors in guinea pig brain membranes. *Neurosci Lett*, **94**, 125–130.

49. Fletcher HP, Noble S and Spratto GR (1989) Effect of the acetylcholinesterase inhibitor, soman, on plasma levels of endorphin and adrenocorticotrophic hormone (ACTH). *Biochem Pharmacol*, **38**, 2045–2046.

50. Fosbraey P, Wetherell JR and French MC (1990) Neurotransmitter changes in guinea-pig brain regions following soman intoxication. *J Neurochem*, **54**, 72–79.

51. Naseem SM (1990) Effect of organophosphates on dopamine and muscarinic receptor binding in rat brain. *Biochem Int*, **20**, 799–806.

52. Smallbridge RC, Carr RE and Fein HG (1991) Diisopropylfluorophosphate (DFP) reduces serum prolactin, thyrotropin, luteinizing hormone, and growth hormone and increases adrenocorticotropic and corticosterone in rats: involvement of dopaminergic and somatostatinergic as well as cholinergic pathways. *Toxicol Appl Pharmacol*, **108**, 284–295.

53. Senanayake N and Karalliedde L (1987) Neurotoxic effects of organophosphorus insecticides. An intermediate syndrome. *N Engl J Med*, **316**, 761–763.

54. Senanayake N and Karalliedde L (1992) The intermediate syndrome in anticholinesterase neurotoxicity. In: *Clinical and Experimental Toxicology of Organophosphates and Carbamates* (B Ballantyne and TC Marrs, eds), pp. 126–134. Oxford: Butterworth-Heinemann.

55. Preusser H-J (1967) Die Ultrastructur der motorischen Endplatte im Zwerchfell der Ratte und Veranderungen nach Inhibierung der Acetylcholinesterase. *Z Zellforsch*, **80**, 436–457.

56. Ariens AT, Wolthuis OL and van Bentham RMJ (1969) Reversible necrosis at the end plate region in striated muscles of the rat poisoned with cholinesterase inhibitors. *Experientia*, **1**, 57–59.

57. Gupta RC, Patterson GT and Dettbarn W-D (1987) Acute tabun toxicity; biochemical and histochemical consequences in brain and skeletal muscles of rats. *Toxicology*, **46**, 329–341.

58. Gupta RC, Patterson GT and Dettbarn W-D (1987) Biochemical and histochemical alterations following acute soman intoxication in the rat. *Toxicol Appl Pharmacol*, **87**, 393–402.

59. Hughes JN, Knight R, Brown RFR and Marrs TC (1991) Effects of experimental sarin intoxication on the morphology of the mouse diaphragm: a light and electron microscopical study. *Int J Exp Pathol*, **72**, 195–209.

60. Leonard JP and Salpeter MM (1979) Agonist induced myopathy at the neuromuscular junction is mediated by calcium. *J Cell Biol*, **82**, 811–819.

61. Marrs TC, Bright JE, Inns RH and Tuckwell NJ (1990) Histochemical demonstration of calcium influx into mouse diaphragms induced by sarin. *Toxicologist*, **10**, 132.

62. Inns RH, Tuckwell NJ, Bright JE and Marrs TC (1990) Histochemical demonstration of calcium accumulation in muscle fibres after experimental organophosphate poisoning. *Human Exp Toxicol*, **9**, 245–250.

63. Johnson MK (1975) Organophosphorus esters causing delayed neurotoxic effects. *Arch Toxicol*, **34**, 259–288.

64. Anderson RJ and Dunham CB (1985) Electrophysiologic changes in peripheral nerve following repeated exposure to organophosphorus agents. *Arch Toxicol*, **58**, 97–101.

65. Johnson MK, Willems JL, de Bisschop HC *et al.* (1985) Can soman cause delayed neuropathy? *Fund Appl Toxicol*, **5**, S180–S181.

66. Parker RM, Crowell JA, Bucci TJ and Dacre JC (1988) Negative delayed neuropathy study in chickens after treatment with isopropyl methylphosphonofluoridate (sarin, type 1). *Toxicologist*, **8**, 248.

67. Henderson JD, Higgins RJ, Dacre JC and Wilson BW (1992) Neurotoxicity of acute and repeated treatments of tabun, paraoxon, diisopropyl fluorophosphate and isofenphos to the hen. *Toxicology*, **72**, 117–129.

68. Gordon JJ, Inns RH, Johnson MK *et al.* (1983) The delayed neuropathic effects of nerve agents and some other organophosphate compounds. *Arch Toxicol*, **51**, 71–82.

69. Aldridge WN, Barnes JM and Johnson MK (1969) Studies on delayed neuropathy produced by some organophosphorus compounds. *Ann NY Acad Sci*, **160**, 314–322.

70. Ludomirsky A, Klein HO and Sarelli P (1982) Q-T prolongations and polymorphous ('torsade de pointes') ventricular arrhythmias associated with organophosphorus insecticide poisoning. *Am J Cardiol*, **49**, 1654–1658.

71. McDonough JH, Jaax NK, Crowley RA *et al.* (1989) Atropine and/or diazepam therapy protects against soman-induced neural and cardiac pathology. *Fund Appl Toxicol*, **13**, 256–276.

72. Pimentel JH and Carrington da Costa RB (1992) Effects of organophosphates on the heart. In: *Clinical and Experimental Toxicology of Organophosphates and Carbamates* (B Ballantyne and TC Marrs, eds), pp. 145–148. Oxford: Butterworth-Heinemann.

73. Brimblecombe RW (1974) *Drug Actions in Cholinergic System*, pp. 64–132. New York: Macmillan.

74. Wolthuis OL and Vanwersch RAP (1984) Behavioral changes in the rat after low doses of cholinesterase inhibitors. *Fund Appl Toxicol*, **4**, S195–S208.

75. McDonough JH, Smith RF and Smith CD (1986) Behavioral correlates of soman-induced neuropathology: deficits in DRL acquisition. *Behav Toxicol Teratol*, **8**, 179–187.

76. Anzueto A, Berdine GG, Moore GT *et al.* (1986) Pathophysiology of soman intoxication in primates. *Toxicol Appl Pharmacol*, **86**, 56–68.

77. McLeod CG (1985) Pathology of nerve agents: perspectives on medical management. *Fund Appl Toxicol*, **5**, S10–S16.

78. Martin LJ, Doebbler JA, Shih T-M and Anthony A (1985) Protective effect of diazepam pretreatment on soman-induced brain lesion formation. *Brain Res*, **325**, 287–289.

79. Petras JM (1981) Soman neurotoxicity. *Fund Appl Toxicol*, **1**, 242.

80. Holmes JH and Gaon MD (1956) Observations on acute and multiple exposure to anticholinesterase agents. *Trans Am Clin Chem Assoc*, **68**, 86–103.
81. Marrs TC and Maynard RL (1994) Neurotoxicity of chemical warfare agents. In: *Handbook of Clinical Neurology* (PJ Vinken, GW Bruyn and FA de Wolff, eds), pp. 233–247. Amsterdam: Elsevier.
82. Korsak RJ and Sato MM (1977) Effects of chronic organophosphate pesticide exposure on the central nervous system. *Clin Toxicol*, **11**, 83–95.
83. Hirshberg A and Lerman Y (1984) Clinical problems in organophosphate poisoning: the use of a computerized information system. *Fund Appl Toxicol*, **4**, S209–S214.
84. Rosenstock L, Keifer M, Daniell WE *et al.* (1991) Chronic central nervous system effects of acute organophosphate pesticide poisoning. *Lancet*, **338**, 223–227.
85. Durham WF, Wolfe HR and Quinby GE (1965) Organophosphorus insecticides and mental alertness. *Arch Environ Health*, **10**, 55–66.
86. Levin HS and Rodnitzky RL (1976) Behavioral effects of organophosphate pesticides in man. *Clin Toxicol*, **9**, 391–405.
87. Rodnitzky RL, Levin HS and Mick DL (1975) Occupational exposure to organophosphate pesticides: a neurobehavioral study. *Arch Environ Health*, **30**, 98–103.
88. Dille JR and Smith PW (1964) Central nervous system effects of chronic exposure to organophosphate insecticides. *Aerospace Med*, **35**, 475–478.
89. Gershon S and Shaw FH (1961) Psychiatric sequelae of chronic exposure to organophosphorus insecticides. *Lancet*, **I**, 1371–1374.
90. Maizlish N, Schenker M, Weisskopf C *et al.* (1987) A behavioral evaluation of pest control workers with short-term low-level exposure to the organophosphate diazinon. *Am J Ind Med*, **12**, 153–172.
91. Duffy FH, Burchfiel JL, Bartels PH *et al.* (1979) Long-term effects of an organophosphate upon the human electroencephalogram. *Toxicol Appl Pharmacol*, **47**, 161–176.
92. Burchfiel JL, Duffy FH and Sim van M (1976) Persistent effects of sarin and dieldrin upon the primate electroencephalogram. *Toxicol Appl Pharmacol*, **35**, 365–379.
93. Masuda N, Takatsu M, Morinari H and Ozawa T (1995) Sarin poisoning on the Tokyo subway. *Lancet*, **345**, 1446.
94. Nozaki H and Aikawa N (1995) Sarin poisoning on the Tokyo subway. *Lancet*, **345**, 1446–1447.

4

TREATMENT AND PROPHYLAXIS OF ORGANOPHOSPHATE NERVE AGENT POISONING

The treatment of organophosphate (OP) nerve agent poisoning is similar in many respects to that used in the treatment of OP insecticide poisoning. On the other hand there are a number of additional challenges such as treatment under suboptimal conditions (the battlefield). In addition, aging (see below) renders the question of prophylaxis and pretreatment important, especially with soman.

As in all cases of poisoning by chemical warfare agents, casualties should be removed as soon as possible from the source of contamination and decontaminated. Contaminated clothing should be removed by staff wearing adequate protective clothing, suitable impermeable gloves and a respirator. Standard procedures for removal of contaminated clothing have been developed in some countries and practice of these drills is essential if removal of clothing is to be rapid and without risk of secondary contamination of the patient. This is particularly the case when dealing with casualties contaminated with thickened nerve agent, e.g. soman.

Under battlefield conditions removal of casualties to an area where decontamination can be practiced may be delayed and the rapid administration of therapy becomes the priority. Details of the drugs in use are provided below. It is noteworthy that auto-injection devices designed to allow the rapid administration of drugs are available. It should be obvious that these devices should be tested under realistic conditions: needles should penetrate protective clothing and standard military dress.

In addition to the need for the rapid administration of drug therapy, other measures will be necessary: thus casualties may suffer from respiratory depression and resuscitation may be necessary. This presents formidable problems on a contaminated battlefield. It should be stressed that there is no case for the person administering first aid removing his or her own respirator and applying mouth-to-mouth artificial respiration. The casualty's respirator may have to be removed, though this will be dangerous if contamination is still present, and artificial respiration applied by means of a bag (Ambu bag) equipped with a suitable filter and covered with protective material. The use of an oropharyngeal airway may be helpful.

If possible, casualties who have stopped breathing should be ventilated with air enriched with oxygen. However, the provision of bottled oxygen on the battlefield is all but impossible, although oxygen concentrator devices can be fitted in field ambulances and used there. Some countries have considered moving oxygen forward in the battle zone: this is a matter of individual national military doctrine.

Once casualties have been removed to an area where decontamination is possible, contaminated clothing should be removed and the casualty put into a clean, protective casualty bag if there is any delay before admission to a clean area for further treatment. Monitoring devices should be used for checking the success of decontamination drills before the casualty is admitted to the clean area. Defense of this clean area is of paramount importance and under no circumstances should inadequately decontaminated casualties be hurried through into this area on the grounds that they are severely injured. Contamination of the clean area will severely endanger the lives of those working in it and hence reduce the chances of successful treatment of future casualties.

ANTIDOTES

The main drugs used in the treatment of nerve gas poisoning are anticholinergics such as atropine, pyridinium oximes such as 2-PAM and central nervous system (CNS) depressants such as diazepam. The actions of atropine and the oximes are synergistic.

Atropine

Atropine is a muscarinic cholinergic antagonist, first isolated from *Atropa belladonna* (deadly nightshade) in 1831. It acts by blocking the effects of the acetylcholine that accumulates at muscarinic sites as a consequence of the anticholinesterase actions of the nerve agents and has little effect at nicotinic sites. Although atropine does not readily cross the blood–brain barrier, the drug has some central ameliorative effects in nerve agent poisoning. That it is capable of crossing the blood–brain barrier to some extent is demonstrated by the CNS effects observed in atropine poisoning.

In overdose, atropine can cause hallucinations, ataxia, tachycardia, dry mouth and dilated pupils.

The efficacy of atropine has been extensively studied in animal models. Most studies have involved the use of more than one antidote, sometimes with carbamate prophylaxis, but Lipp[1] showed that atropine alone reversed soman-induced respiratory depression in monkeys. In multiple-antidote studies, usually involving atropine, an oxime, and possibly diazepam and carbamate pretreatment, it appears that atropine and oxime treatment are synergistic and that addition of diazepam confers further benefit. In the case of soman, carbamate prophylaxis confers yet more benefit. However, the conclusion that atropine and oxime act synergistically is a generalization and some studies have shown a more complex interaction between the drugs. Thus Carter et al.[2] showed that, in the guinea pig, atropine and oxime only acted together beneficially at high soman doses and that, at low soman doses, atropine alone was the optimal treatment.

Treatment of nerve agent poisoning with atropine should be instituted as a matter of urgency at a dose of 2 mg intravenously or, less desirably, intramuscularly. The dose should be repeated at 10–15-min intervals. Although plasma atropine levels can be measured, as can cholinesterase levels, neither relates directly to any clinical response and cannot, of course, be performed in the field. The adequacy of dosing with atropine has therefore to be judged by its effects. One might expect reversal of miosis to be a reliable sign of success of treatment with atropine but this is not the case. Nerve-agent-induced miosis is resistant to parenterally administered atropine. Reversal of bradycardia and the drying of salivary secretions are more reliable signs. As a rule of thumb, dosing with atropine should be continued until the heart rate is over 90 beats per minute.

The drying effect of atropine on bronchial secretions may make their removal more difficult and suction may become necessary as a result. In excessive doses, atropine may render the myocardium, particularly if it is hypoxic, excitable and produce arrhythmias. ECG monitoring should be undertaken if at all possible. Overdose can produce hallucinations, anxiety or delirium, together with bladder dysfunction which may necessitate catheterization.

In some cases of OP pesticide poisoning enormous doses of atropine have been used, but in nerve agent poisoning doses above 30 mg are unlikely to be required.

Other anticholinergic drugs have been studied in nerve agent poisoning, for example aprophen, hyoscine, adiphenine and caramiphen: thus Anderson et al.[3] found scopolamine effective against soman-induced incapacitation of guinea pigs; this muscarinic antagonist is also effective against soman-induced convulsions and pathological changes in animals.

Oximes

The pyridinium oximes are divided into the mono- and bispyridinium oximes (Table 1). The main action of the oximes is to reactivate the enzyme acetylcholinesterase by removing the dialkylphosphoryl moiety from the enzyme. In addition, some data exist that show that oximes have beneficial direct effects, including those on ion channels.[4,5] Numerous studies have been carried out into the efficacy of oximes in different species, usually in combination with other drugs, particularly atropine. Thus pralidoxime has been shown to be effective in sarin-poisoned mice, rats, rabbits and dogs.[6–8] Pralidoxime is also effective in VX poisoning in rats.[9] Because of the phenomenon of aging, pralidoxime is not effective in soman poisoning, and

Table 1 Oximes used in the treatment of OP poisoning

Type of oxime	Name	Supplier
Monopyridinium	Pralidoxime chloride (2-PAM) (Protopam chloride)	Ayerst
	Pralidoxime methylsulfate (Contrathion)	SERB
	Pralidoxime methanesulfonate (P2S)	UK government
	Pyrimidoxime	
Bispyridinium	Trimedoxime (TMB-4)	
	Obidoxime (Toxogonin)	Merck
	HI-6	
	HS-6	
	HLö-7	

for different reasons (the nucleophilic attack of pralidoxime is inefficacious) is of little use in tabun poisoning.

Many animal efficacy studies of the bispyridinium oximes have been carried out. Thus obidoxime was shown to be effective in poisoning by sarin[10] and it is also of use, unlike pralidoxime, in tabun poisoning.[11]

The question of which oxime to use is an area of some controversy and disagreement. The choice is mainly between the monopyridinium pralidoxime salts, which are almost certainly equieffective at similar molar doses. Four pralidoxime salts are commercially available, the chloride, the methanesulfonate, the methylsulfate and the methiodide, as is the bispyridinium oxime, obidoxime (Table 1). Obidoxime's noteworthy advantage over the pralidoxime salts, in that obidoxime is effective in animal models in tabun poisoning, has already been mentioned. On the other hand, there has been some concern about the toxicity of obidoxime to the liver, and the significance of this in the choice of oxime is currently unresolved.[12-14]

In addition to pralidoxime salts and obidoxime, the bispyridinium Hagedorn (H) oximes, particularly HI-6, HLö-7, HGG-12 and HGG-42, as well as the monopyridinium oxime pyrimidoxime, have been studied mostly in a military context.[15-17] HI-6 may be beneficial in poisoning with soman, which gives rise to a rapidly aging complex with acetylcholinesterase (see Chapter 3). Some bispyridinium non-oximes such as SAD 128, P-65 and bis(pyridinium-1-methyl) ether, have some activity in soman poisoning,[11] and the effect of HI-6 is possibly a similar and direct pharmacological action of the oxime.[18] It has, however, been reported that HI-6 may reactivate aged soman-inhibited acetylcholinesterase.[19,20] Nevertheless, this probably only applies to peripheral acetylcholinesterase and to unaged soman-inhibited enzyme. Limited civilian use in organophosphorus pesticide poisoning in the former Yugoslavia suggests that HI-6 might represent an improvement on its predecessors.[21] Like pralidoxime, HI-6 is not very effective in tabun poisoning, but the novel Hagedorn oxime HLö-7 appears to have reactivating potency for both soman- and tabun-inhibited cholinesterase and thus may represent a universal OP antidote!

The search for oximes which can reverse the effects of soman poisoning continues in a number of laboratories. It should be recalled that once aging of the agent–enzyme complex is established it is unlikely that any oxime will be effective. Aging of the soman–enzyme complex occurs rapidly (Chapter 3), and early treatment remains vital.

The use of oximes such as HI-6 and HLö-7 presents practical difficulties for military authorities. These oximes are not stable in aqueous solution and thus a more complex auto-injection device than that used to deliver pralidoxime or obidoxime would be needed. Such devices are referred to as 'wet–dry' auto-injection devices, and although development is well advanced and such devices are commercially available, they are more costly than the simpler devices. Before HI-6 can be administered from an auto-injection device, mixing of the solute and solvent is required and it may be that this will delay, if only briefly, the administration of the drug. Whether this will be important under field conditions has not yet been determined.

A number of non-pharmacological points are important in the design of devices intended for issue to troops. Devices may well need to be stockpiled against the risk of war and they should be stable for a number of years. Storage conditions should not be too demanding and the devices should be proof against a certain amount of mishandling under battlefield conditions: optimal storage will probably not be available.

Until a few years ago, it was generally accepted that oxime treatment should be stopped quite early in OP poisoning. More recently, the tendency, at least with pesticides, has been to advise longer treatment. However, before longer treatment protocols are adopted for nerve agents, it should be remembered that toxicokinetics is an area where OP pesticides and nerve agents may differ considerably.

The toxicity of oximes is unlikely to be a problem in clinical use. The bispyridinium oxime, TBM-4, is notably more toxic than the others and the possible hepatotoxicity of obidoxime has been discussed above. Some oximes, for example diisonitrosoacetone, are cyanogenic. However, the toxicity of P2S is not, to any substantial degree, caused by cyanogenesis.[22] Nevertheless, if injected too rapidly, P2S can cause nausea, dizziness, tachycardia, hyperventilation and muscle weakness. Intramuscular P2S causes local muscle necrosis and, given orally, the drug causes gastrointestinal upset. For a review of the toxicology of oximes see Marrs.[14]

ProPAM, the tertiary amine analog of pralidoxime, penetrates the CNS more readily than pralidoxime. Consequently, ProPAM would be expected to have a greater beneficial effect in nerve agent poisoning than pralidoxime. This expectation has not in general been realized in experimental studies.

The aim of therapy with pralidoxime salts has traditionally been to maintain plasma concentrations > 4 mg l^{-1}. To this end the methanesulfonate should be given by slow intravenous injection or, less ideally, intramuscularly at a dose of 500 mg to 1 g. Dosing with pralidoxime methanesulfonate should be repeated at 15-min intervals up to a total dose of 2 g (30 mg kg^{-1}) or, in extreme circumstances, 4 g. During treatment the patient's status should be monitored for side-effects of oximes. If the chloride of pralidoxime is used, the dose should be adjusted for the different molecular weight. It should be noted that recommended doses of the methylsulfate are somewhat lower, although, on a molar basis, this drug is likely to be equieffective with the other two salts: the reason for the discrepancy is unclear. In the Tokyo sarin incident, pralidoxime methiodide was used. Obidoxime may be used in tabun poisoning but neither pralidoxime salts nor obidoxime are likely to be effective in soman poisoning.

Central nervous system depressants

Diazepam is of benefit in reducing apprehension, agitation and muscular fasciculation and in stopping convulsions.[23,24] Midazolam and, as an anticonvulsant, phenytoin are possible alternatives,[25] as is the centrally active antimuscarinic benactyzine[26] (Table 2).

Anticonvulsants, including diazepam, were first studied for the treatment of organophosphate-induced convulsions on the empirical basis that they were effective in other types of convulsions. In view of the possibility, previously discussed in Chapter 3, that convulsions are likely to have long-term deleterious effects on the CNS, this aspect of nerve agent therapy is clearly of importance and indeed it appears that histological changes produced in the central nervous systems of rats by injection of just sublethal doses of soman can be prevented with diazepam.[30] The other main use of diazepam is in the prevention or amelioration of muscle fasciculations.

Despite the introduction of diazepam as a symptomatic anticonvulsant, a number of studies have been performed which indicate that the effects of diazepam may be more specific. These studies have mainly investigated the effect on cholinergic and GABAergic systems, as well as cGMP levels. Thus Tonkapii et al.[32] showed that diazepam, 20 mg kg^{-1}, increased the acetylcholine content of mouse brain, while in rat corpus striatum and hippocampus, diazepam decreased elevations in choline levels produced by sarin and soman, but not those of acetylcholine.[33] Lundgren et

Table 2 Anticonvulsants studied for the possible treatment of nerve agent poisoning

Drug group	Drug	Reference
Benzodiazepines	Diazepam	Lipp[23,24]
	Clonazepam	Lipp[27]
Barbiturates	Phenobarbitone	Kleinrok and Jagiello-Wojtowicz[28]
	Pentobarbitone	Dretchen et al.[29]
Hydantoins	Phenytoin	Kleinrok and Jagiello-Wojtowicz[28]
Local anesthetics		Klemm[31]
Ca^{2+} channel blockers		Dretchen et al.[29]

al.[34] suggested that diazepam might have an effect on choline transport across the blood–brain barrier as well as on acetylcholine turnover. Whether the effects of diazepam on the GABAergic system underlay the anticonvulsant activity of the drug in soman poisoning has not been resolved.[35] Lundy and Magor[36] hypothesized an effect on soman-induced elevations in central nervous cGMP levels as a mechanism of action of the benzodiazepines, while there is some evidence for beneficial activity on the peripheral nervous system in OP poisoning.[37]

Studies have shown that an anticonvulsive effect of diazepam is obtained at plasma levels of 400–500 μg l^{-1} or above.[38]

Most experimental work on the efficacy of diazepam in OP poisoning has been carried out using treatment combinations, usually diazepam, atropine and oximes, and sometimes with carbamate pretreatment. Thus Lipp[23,24] showed that diazepam and atropine in combination was more effective than atropine alone in soman poisoning of monkeys, while anticonvulsant activity was demonstrated in soman-poisoned rats by Churchill *et al.*[39] Rump and Grudzinska[40] showed that diazepam, with atropine and obidoxime, substantially raised the LD$_{50}$ of diisopropyl phosphorofluoridate (DFP) in rats. A combination of atropine and diazepam has been shown to be effective in poisoning with tabun, sarin and VX, as well as soman, after carbamate pretreatment, in guinea pigs.[11] Thus diazepam seems to have a broad spectrum of activity against chemical warfare agents. However, there is little evidence of much benefit from diazepam alone in the treatment of OP poisoning, although some studies have shown a minor beneficial effect, for example after pretreatment with diazepam alone in soman poisoning of rabbits.[37] At certain doses of nerve agent, the use of diazepam may contribute to the incapacitation produced,[3] but this is a price to be paid for its generally beneficial activity.

The effect of drugs recommended in the treatment of nerve agent poisoning on the fighting performance of soldiers in the field has been suggested to be a problem. In practice the soldiers exposed to nerve agent and who develop symptoms and signs which suggest that therapy is necessary are unlikely to take much further part in the immediate military action. A more likely problem is presented by the inappropriate administration of therapy, e.g. auto-injection devices, by soldiers who have not actually been exposed to nerve agent. Whether such administration would be common under battlefield conditions is a matter of discipline and training in the recognition of the early signs of nerve agent poisoning. The effects of inappropriate administration of therapy may be anticipated to be dose dependent. Inappropriate administration of 2 mg of atropine will lead to some deterioration in performance, though it might be expected that the individuals could continue with their duties, while inappropriate administration of 4 mg of atropine would have a serious effect on performance. Inappropriate administration of 6 mg of atropine would be likely to incapacitate the individual concerned. The additional effects of the oxime and possibly diazepam would, if anything, add to these effects, though it is likely that the effects of atropine would predominate.

The administration of diazepam on the battlefield under conditions when full protective clothing is being worn presents serious difficulties. Auto-injection devices issued to UK forces until recently carried a 5-mg diazepam tablet in a detachable cap. The tablet was to be swallowed. Of course, to do this the respirator would have to be temporarily lifted, and training to ensure that this can be done rapidly and safely is necessary. More recently a lysine–diazepam conjugate has been included with atropine and P2S in the auto-injection devices. The removal of the need to take diazepam by mouth is a major step forward in the treatment of nerve agent poisoning under battlefield conditions. For treatment, diazepam (5 mg) should be administered intravenously: this should be done as soon as the casualty has been decontaminated and transferred to a clean environment. The dose may be repeated at 15-min intervals up to a maximum of 15 mg.

Calcium-channel blockers

Calcium-channel blockers, such as verapamil, nifedipine, nitrendipine and nimopedine, have been shown to be effective against the lethal effects of OPs such as DFP and soman in animal models. This effect appears to be independent of the anticonvulsant properties of these drugs[41] and these drugs may, in the future, have a role in the treatment of OP poisoning.

COURSE AND PROGNOSIS

Most of the symptoms and clinical signs of OP nerve poisoning are potentially reversible. However, there is recognition that survival after high doses of OPs (and possibly lower doses) may result in long-term effects upon the CNS. It is unlikely that nerve agents possess the potential to give rise to organophosphate-induced delayed neuropathy.

The prognosis for the poisoned soldier is almost inevitably worse than that for a poisoned civilian: treatment may be delayed and less adequate. Soldiers who are caught unawares and who are exposed to large doses of nerve agent before donning respirators and other protective clothing and who rapidly develop severe symptoms and signs are unlikely to survive. Those who slip rapidly into respiratory failure and who become incapable of self-administering their own auto-injection devices will also have a poor prognosis unless help is rapidly provided. Casualties arriving at first aid posts, or better at field hospitals, still breathing and with adequate therapy already instituted have a good chance of survival.

SPECIFIC PROBLEMS WITH PARTICULAR NERVE AGENTS

Sarin and VX

Therapy with atropine (2 mg at 15-min intervals until atropinization is achieved) should be started. P2S (500 mg by slow intravenous injection at 15-min intervals up to 2 g in total) should be given. Diazepam 5 mg by slow intravenous injection should be given, up to a maximum dose at 15 mg. More may be given if convulsions occur.

Atropine eye drops had some beneficial effects on the eye signs and symptoms observed in the Tokyo sarin incident, but at the price of impaired accommodation.

Tabun

Atropine and diazepam should be given as with sarin and VX. P2S is not very effective at reactivating the tabun–acetylcholinesterase complex (see above), so the oxime of choice with this nerve agent is obidoxime. The dose should be 250 mg by slow intravenous infusion. Diazepam should be given as above.

Soman

The rapid aging (monodealkylation) of soman-inhibited acetylcholinesterase has already been discussed. This prevents both spontaneous reactivation and reactivation induced by oximes, with the possible exception of some of the Hagedorn oximes. Nevertheless, atropine is still effective and should be given (see above), as should diazepam. The only other approach likely to be successful is prophylaxis (see below).

PROPHYLAXIS OF NERVE AGENT POISONING

As was discussed in Chapter 3, treatment of soman poisoning is difficult because of the rapid aging of the complex formed when soman inhibits acetylcholinesterase. This has made the idea of prophylaxis attractive. However, prophylaxis may have attractions even against more readily treatable nerve agent poisoning. It might, for example, effectively raise the minimum incapacitating dose of nerve agent. A number of compounds have been studied with a view to prophylaxis (Table 3). Of these, the carbamates, physostigmine and pyridostigmine, have been most widely studied and seem most promising.

There has been debate amongst those involved in the development of ways of managing nerve agent poisoning regarding the terms prophylaxis and pretreatment. It has come to be accepted that the pre-poisoning administration of drugs which enhance the likely efficacy of post-poisoning therapy is described as pretreatment. The pre-poisoning administration of drugs which render post-poisoning therapy unnecessary is described as prophylaxis. Carbamates such as pyridostigmine bromide are used as pretreatment.

Carbamates

In 1946 Koster[42] showed that the carbamate anticholinesterase physostigmine could protect cat cholinesterase against inactivation by DFP *in vivo*, and in the same year Koelle[43] demonstrated that physostigmine or neostigmine could protect cholinesterase against inactivation by DFP *in vitro*. The action of the carbamates is dependent on the fact that they form complexes with cholinesterase which are refractory to

Table 3 Substances used experimentally or clinically in the prophylaxis of nerve agent poisoning

Mode of action	Drug group	Drug
Protect enzyme	Carbamates	Physostigmine
		Pyridostigmine
		Mobam
		Decarbofuran
	Aminophenols	Eseroline
	Organophosphates	TEPP
		Paraoxon
		Ethyl 4-nitrophenyl methylphosphonate
Anticholinergics	Antimuscarinic	Atropine
		Aprophen
		Hyoscine
		Adiphenine
		Caramiphen
	Antinicotinic	Pentamethonium
		Mecamylamine
Neuromuscular blockers		d-Tubocurarine
Enzyme reactivators	Oximes	Pralidoxime salts
		Obidoxime
		HI-6
CNS depressants	Diazepam	
	Clonazepam	
Acetylcholinesterase Monoclonal antibodies against OPs		

phosphorylation but which decarbamylate (and therefore reactivate) spontaneously and rapidly. Berry and Davies[44] showed in guinea pigs that physostigmine could substantially raise the LD_{50} of soman. Investigators have studied a number of carbamates in nerve agent prophylaxis, but the most important are pyridostigmine and physostigmine. The work of Inns and Leadbeater[11] showed clearly that, at least in guinea pigs, the optimum combined therapy was combined pretreatment with a carbamate (pyridostigmine) and post-poisoning therapy with atropine, pralidoxime mesylate and diazepam. The pretreatment dosage is pyridostigmine bromide 30 mg orally every 8 h.

Under field conditions pyridostigmine bromide tablets (30 mg) are administered every 8 h. Satisfactory blood levels of pyridostigmine are achieved rapidly, and by about the third dose inhibition of red cell cholinesterase will have stabilized at about 20%. Some side-effects may be expected, including, in some individuals, diarrhea. Of course, the inappropriate administration of more than the recommended dose will lead to more severe side-effects and, again, good discipline is necessary to ensure correct dosing: the idea that if one tablet helps, three all at once should produce complete safety, should be dispelled.

OPs

Oxime-responsive OPs, i.e. those whose OP–cholinesterase complex does not age, can theoretically also be used as soman prophylaxis. In this context Berry et al.[45] studied TEPP (tetraethylpyrophosphate), paraoxon and ethyl 4-nitrophenyl methyl-phosphonate.

Other prophylaxes

Most other drugs studied in nerve agent prophylaxis are more familiar as post-poisoning antidotes. Anticholinergics such as atropine have been studied, as well as CNS depressants. At one time the UK armed forces were issued with P2S tablets as pretreatment: the theory is that they would act before any substantial proportion of the enzyme ages. Another approach to the prophylaxis of nerve agent poisoning has been the use of exogenous acetylcholinesterase or butyrylcholinesterase. In view of the very high affinity of nerve agents for cholinesterase, the use of exogenous enzyme is a logical approach. Bovine fetal serum acetylcholinesterase can protect mice against many multiples of the LD_{50} of nerve agents. This treatment has only reached an experimental stage, but with the advent of biotechnology, logistical problems with enzyme treatment might be overcome.

REFERENCES

1. Lipp JA (1976) Effects of atropine upon the cardiovascular system during coma induced respiratory depression. *Arch Int Pharmacodyn*, **220**, 19–27.
2. Carter WH, Jones DE and Carchman RA (1985) Application of response surface methods for evaluating the interactions of soman, atropine and pralidoxime chloride. *Fund Appl Toxicol*, **5**, 5232–5241.
3. Anderson DR, Gennings C, Carter WH et al. (1994) Efficacy of scopolamine and diazepam against soman-induced debilitation in guinea pigs. *Fund Appl Toxicol*, **22**, 588–593.
4. Alkonden M, Rao KS and Albuquerque EX (1988) Acetylcholinesterase reactivators modify the functional properties of the nicotine acetylcholine receptor ion channel. *J Pharmacol Exp Ther*, **245**, 543–556.
5. Reddy VK, Deshpande SS, Cintra WM et al. (1991) Effectiveness of oximes 2-PAM and HI-6 in recovery of muscle function depressed by organophosphate agents in the rat hemidiaphragm: an *in vitro* study. *Fund Appl Toxicol*, **17**, 746–760.
6. Davies DR, Green HL and Willey GL (1959) 2-Hydroxyiminomethyl-N-methylpyridi-nium methanesulphonate and atropine in the treatment of severe organophosphate poisoning. *Br J Pharmacol*, **14**, 5–8.
7. Crook JW, Goodman AI and Colbourne JL (1962) Adjunctive value of oral prophylaxis with the oximes 2-PAM lactate and 2-PAM methanesulfonate to therapeutic administra-

tion of atropine in dogs poisoned by inhaled sarin vapour. *J Pharmacol Exp Ther*, **136**, 397–399.

8. Johnson DD and Stewart WC (1970) The effects of atropine, pralidoxime and lidocaine on nerve–muscle and respiratory function in organophosphate-treated rabbits. *Can J Physiol Pharmacol*, **48**, 625–630.

9. Harris LW and Stitcher DL (1983) Reactivation of VX-inhibited cholinesterase by 2-PAM and HS-6 in rats. *Drug Chem Toxicol*, **6**, 235–240.

10. Borbely AA, Tunod U and Hopft W (1975) Studies on the protective action of atropine and obidoxime against sarin poisoning in mice. In: *Cholinergic Mechanisms* (PG Waser, ed.), pp. 427–432. New York: Raven Press.

11. Inns RH and Leadbeater L (1983) The efficacy of bispyridinium derivatives in the treatment of organophosphate poisoning in the guinea-pig. *J Pharm Pharmacol*, **35**, 427–433.

12. von Bisa K, Fischer G, Muller O *et al.* (1964) Die Antidotwirkung von Bis-(4-hydroxyiminomethyl-pyridinium methyl)-äther-dichlorid bei mit Alkylphosphat vergifteten Ratten. *Arzneimittelforsch*, **14**, 85–88.

13. Wirth W (1968) Schadigungsmöglichkeiten durch Antidot. *Arch Toxikol*, **24**, 71–82.

14. Marrs TC (1991) Toxicology of oximes used in the treatment of organophosphate poisoning. *Adverse Drug React Acute Pois Rev*, **10**, 61–73.

15. Bismuth C, Inns RH and Marrs TC (1992) Efficacy, toxicity and clinical use of oximes in anticholinesterase poisoning. In: *Clinical and Experimental Toxicology of Organophosphates and Carbamates* (B Ballantyne and TC Marrs, eds), pp. 555–577. Oxford: Butterworth-Heinemann.

16. van Helden HPM, van der Wiel HJ, Zijlstra JJ *et al.* (1994) Comparison of the therapeutic effects and pharmacokinetics of HI-6, HLö-7, HGG-12, HGG-42 and obidoxime following non-reactivatable acetylcholinesterase inhalation in rats. *Arch Toxicol*, **68**, 224–236.

17. Worek F, Kirchner T and Sczinicz L (1994) Treatment of tabun poisoned guinea-pigs with atropine HLö-7 or HI-6: effect on respiratory and circulating function. *Arch Toxicol*, **68**, 231–239.

18. Clement JG and Lockwood PA (1982) HI-6, an oxime which is an effective antidote of soman poisoning; a structure activity study. *Toxicol Appl Pharmacol*, **64**, 140–146.

19. Shih T-M, Whalley CE and Valdes JP (1991) A comparison of cholinergic effects of HI-6 and pralidoxime-2-chloride (2-PAM) in soman poisoning. *Toxicol Lett*, **55**, 131–147.

20. Shih T-M (1993) Comparison of several oximes on reactivation of soman inhibited blood, brain and tissue cholinesterase activity in rats. *Arch Toxicol*, **67**, 637–646.

21. Kusić R, Jovanović D, Randjelović S *et al.* (1991) HI-6 in man: efficacy of the oxime in poisoning by organophosphate insecticides. *Human Exp Toxicol*, **10**, 113–118.

22. Enander I, Sundwall A and Sörbo B (1961) Metabolic studies on N-methylpyridinium-2-aldoxime 1. The conversion to thiocyanate. *Biochem Pharmacol*, **7**, 226–231.

23. Lipp JA (1972) Effect of diazepam upon soman-induced seizure activity and convulsions. *Electroencephalogr Clin Neurophysiol*, **32**, 557–560.

24. Lipp JA (1973) Effect of benzodiazepine derivatives on soman-induced seizure activity and convulsions in the monkey. *Arch Int Pharmacodyn*, **202**, 244–251.

25. Sellström Å (1992) Anticonvulsants in anticholinesterase poisoning. In: *Clinical and Experimental Toxicology of Organophosphates and Carbamates* (B Ballantyne and TC Marrs, eds), pp. 578–586. Oxford: Butterworth-Heinemann.

26. Hauser W, Kirsch DM and Weger N (1981) Therapeutic effects of new oximes, benactyzine and atropine in soman poisoning. Part II: effect of HGG-12, HGG-42 and obidoxime in poisoning with various anticholinesterase agents in beagle dogs. *Fund Appl Toxicol*, **1**, 164–168.

27. Lipp JA (1974) Effect of small doses of clonazenam upon soman-induced seizure activity and convulsions. *Arch Int Pharmacodyn Ther*, **210**, 49–54.

28. Kleinrok Z and Jagiełło-Wojtowicz E (1977) The influence of some anticonvulsant drugs on the acute toxicity of diisopropylfluorophosphate in mice. *Ann Univ Mariae Sklodowska Med*, **32**, 155–160.

29. Dretchen KI, Bowles HM and Raines A (1986) Protection by phenytoin and calcium channel blocking agents against the toxicity of diisopropylphosphorofluoridate. *Toxicol Appl Pharmacol*, **83**, 584–589.

30. Martin LJ, Doebler JA and Shih TM (1985) Protective effect of diazepam pretreatment on soman-induced brain lesion formation. *Brain Res*, **325**, 287–289.

31. Klemm WR (1985) Comparison of known sodium-channel blockers in DFP toxicity. *Toxicol Lett*, **25**, 307–312.

32. Tonkopii VD, Sofronov GA, Aleksanriiskaya IE and Brestkina LM (1978) Mechanism of the action of diazepam on the brain acetylcholine level in mice. *Byull Eksperim Biol Medit*, **86**, 38–49.

33. Flynn CJ and Wecker L (1986) Elevated choline levels in brain: a noncholinergic component of organophosphate toxicity. *Biochem Pharmacol*, **35**, 3115–3122.

34. Lundgren G, Nordgren I and Karlen B (1987) Effect of diazepam pretreatment on blood choline and acetylcholine turnover in brain of mice. *Pharmacol Toxicol*, **67**, 69–99.

35. Lundy PM, Magor G and Shaw RK (1978) Gamma aminobutyric acid metabolism in different areas of rat brain at the onset of soman-induced convulsions. *Arch Int Pharmacodyn*, **234**, 64–73.

36. Lundy PM and Magor G (1978) Cyclic GMP concentrations in cerebellum following organophosphate administration. *J Pharm Pharmacol*, **30**, 251–252.

37. Johnson DD and Lowndes HE (1974) Reduction by diazepam of repetitive electrical activity and toxicity resulting from soman. *Eur J Pharmacol*, **28**, 245–250.

38. Hvidberg EF and Dam M (1976) Clinical pharmacokinetics of anticonvulsants. *Clin Pharmacokin*, **1**, 161–188.

39. Churchill L, Padzernik TL, Cross RS *et al.* (1987) Cholinergic systems influence local cerebral glucose use in specific anatomical areas: DFP versus soman. *Neuroscience*, **20**, 329–340.

40. Rump S and Grudzinska E (1974) Investigations on the effects of local anaesthetics in organic phosphate intoxication. *Arch Int Pharmacodyn Ther*, **182**, 178–181.

41. Dretchen KI, Henderson TR and Raines A (1992) Calcium channel blocking agents in the management of acute cholinesterase poisoning. In: *Clinical and Experimental Toxicology of Organophosphates and Carbamates* (B Ballantyne and TC Marrs, eds), pp. 587–595. Oxford: Butterworth-Heinemann.

42. Koster R (1946) Synergisms and antagonisms between physostigmine and diisopropyl fluorophosphate in cats. *J Pharmacol Exp Ther*, **88**, 39–46.

43. Koelle GB (1946) Protection of cholinesterase against irreversible inactivation by DFP *in vitro*. *J Pharmacol Exp Ther*, **88**, 323–327.

44. Berry WK and Davies DR (1970) The use of carbamates and atropine in the protection of animals against poisoning by 1,2,2-trimethylpropyl methyl phosphonofluoridate. *Biochem Pharmacol*, **19**, 927–934.

45. Berry WK, Davies DR and Gordon JJ (1971) Protection of animal against soman (1,2,2-trimethylpropyl methylphosphonofluoridate) by pretreatment with some other organophosphorus compounds, followed by oxime and atropine. *Biochem Pharmacol*, **20**, 125–134.

5

A HISTORY OF HUMAN STUDIES WITH NERVE AGENTS BY THE UK AND USA

The views expressed in this chapter are those of the author and should not be construed as the position or policy of the Department of the Army (USA) unless so designated by other authorized documents.

INTRODUCTION

The toxic organophosphorus cholinesterase-inhibiting substances that are known as nerve agents were first synthesized by a German chemist, Dr Gerhard Schrader, in 1936. Germany manufactured and stockpiled two of these compounds, tabun (GA) and sarin (GB), and developed a third, soman (GD), during World War II. Since the Allies had no knowledge of these agents and no defense against them, it was fortunate that Germany did not use them. Organophosphorus cholinesterase inhibitors were first synthesized in the mid-1800s, but were not used as warfare agents. In fact, English officials had studied and rejected one, diisopropyl phosphorofluoridate (DFP), as a potential chemical agent in the World War II period.

In the closing days of the war in Europe, the USSR captured a manufacturing facility in eastern Germany and moved the facility and personnel to Russia to continue production.[1] In western Germany, the British and the Americans captured a stockpile of munitions containing an unknown chemical agent. Their initial lack of awareness of the properties of this agent, tabun, was indicated in an early British report:

Before the substance was identified, 1 mm. and 2 mm. drops were placed on the skin of the arms of human observers to ascertain whether or not it was a vesicant. The results were negative. A 1 mm. drop was also placed in the eye of a rabbit to show whether the substance caused eye damage. The rabbit went into convulsions and died in a few minutes.[2]

This report also described the first of many studies in animals which were conducted before humans were next exposed to these agents.

The potency of the vapor of these compounds was probably noted by Dr Schrader and his staff, since some reports suggest that they had miosis, eye and head discomfort and dyspnea while working with the substances. Before they realized the volatility and potency of tabun, which was the first agent studied, British scientists also suffered miosis and eye and head discomfort (K. W. Wilson, personal communication).

Beginning at the conclusion of World War II in Europe, the US and the UK military establishments began large research and development programs to investigate the effects of nerve agents and to develop them for military use. Human studies formed an integral part of these programs. This chapter is intended to provide a history of these human studies. However, it is incomplete. Some reports are not easily found and have undoubtedly been overlooked. A few are still classified and cannot be quoted or referenced directly. However, the classified documents contain no significant data that are not also found in the unclassified reports. Finally, this is intended to be a history of a program, not a scientific review of this literature or a description of the clinical effects of nerve agents in humans, reports of which can be found elsewhere.[3]

In the USA, this work was performed under the direct supervision of the Office of The Surgeon General of the Army. For each study a detailed protocol was written and approved by a medical review board which was chaired by a direct appointee of the Surgeon General. A physician prepared to administer emergency care was present during all studies (although he often was not the investigator). Each agent was thoroughly studied by several routes of administration in at least seven species of animals before it was given to humans. Representatives of outside agencies, e.g. the Food and Drug Administration, reviewed the program on several occasions and reported that procedures and standards exceeded those of many other laboratories performing human studies. In the great majority of the studies mentioned, the subjects were enlisted military personnel. In all instances, these personnel volunteered for the studies without coercion and gave informed consent. The conditions under which studies were performed in Great Britain were similar if not identical to those in the USA.

Several initial studies will be mentioned in chronological order. Later studies generally addressed a specific aspect of human pharmacology and these will be discussed by topic. The agent VX was synthesized long after studies on the G agents were underway, and its effects were investigated much later. The first section of this chapter discusses studies with the G agents, the second describes studies with VX, and the third provides an overview of accidental exposures.

G AGENTS

General studies

In the first study,[4] reported in the mid-1940s, 49 subjects were exposed to tabun vapor at Cts of 0.7–21 mg min m^{-3} (one subject with respiratory protection and one eye protected was exposed to a Ct of 30 mg min m^{-3}). (Ct is the product of concentration of vapor or aerosol and time of exposure (mg m^{-3} × min = mg min m^{-3}).) The effects included miosis, frontal headache, retrobulbar pain, engorgement of vessels in the eye, rhinorrhea, nausea and vomiting, and complaints of tightness in the chest and blurring of vision. The signs and symptoms were at their maximal at 24–48 h after exposure. No changes in near or far visual acuity were noted at Cts under 30 mg min m^{-3}. Topical atropine in the eye relieved most of the symptoms, including the nausea and vomiting.

This was followed by a study in which 22 infantry soldiers, 2 officers and 5 civilian scientists were exposed to a Ct of 28 mg min m^{-3} of tabun vapor.[5] The soldiers then performed a number of military field tasks at 2, 5, 24 and 30 h after exposure and also at twilight (about 10 h after exposure). These tasks included assembling and disassembling weapons, shooting a rifle, map reading, use of the compass and slide rule, and writing messages. The scientists performed their usual work. All 29 had miosis, disturbances of vision, and headache; these effects were most severe at 24 h. Of the 29, 22 vomited, 24 had poor or no sleep, 22 had tiredness or lassitude, and 26 felt depressed. Their average far vision changed from 6/6 (meters) before exposure to 6/24 (m) and recovered gradually over a week. Rhinorrhea was common, but there is no mention of lower airway complaints. The conclusions were that the agent produced general harassing effects which would cause some military disability, especially if sustained effort were involved, and that the agent is detectable by eye signs, respiratory effects, and smell. The miosis was felt to be of relatively little importance 'from a practical point of view'. Topical atropine helped vision, gave a large measure of relief, and improved the general well-being of the subjects.

A similar study with GB followed.[6] Subjects received Cts of 3.3 or 6.6 mg min m^{-3} and had miosis and head and eye complaints. Respiratory symptoms were not consistent. When the subjects received a Ct of 3.3 mg min m^{-3} daily for 3 or 4 consecutive days, the eye effects intensified.

A total of 120 subjects were exposed to sarin vapor at Cts of 1, 2, 4 or 6 mg min m^{-3}.[7] At each Ct the time and concentration were changed by a factor of 10; for example, at a Ct of 6 mg min m^{-3} the concentrations were 3.0 and 0.3 mg m^{-3} and the times 2 and 20 min respectively. Rhinorrhea was the most commonly noted effect and occurred in all who received a Ct of 2 mg min m^{-3} or higher. Miosis was noted in all at a Ct of 6 mg min m^{-3}, but was an inconsistent finding at lower Cts. The complaint of a tight chest was more common at Cts of 2 and 4 than at 6 mg min m^{-3}. At the highest Ct, the mean erythrocyte cholinesterase activity after exposure was 73% of the subjects' baseline values for those exposed for 20 min and 87% for those exposed for 2 min.

Eight subjects who inhaled sarin vapor while at rest and nine who inhaled it while exercising had normal neuromuscular function, respiratory function, electrocardiographs and blood cholinesterase after exposure.[8] The retained amount of sarin ranged from 0.16 to 0.8 μg kg^{-1} in the resting group and from 0.29 to 0.99 μg kg^{-1} in the exercising group.

In an attempt to relate erythrocyte cholinesterase activity to signs and symptoms, five subjects received a Ct of 6.6 mg min m^{-3} in a single exposure, and five received two exposures to a Ct of 3.3 mg min m^{-3} 2 or 3 days apart.[9] The first group had miosis and eye symptoms, tight chests, and rhinorrhea. The two-exposure group had fewer effects after the second exposure, and no cumulative effects were noted. In no subject was the erythrocyte cholinesterase activity beyond his normal range (of five samples before the exposure). This was the first of many observations that there is no relationship between the effects caused by direct contact of the nerve agent vapor (on the eye, nose and airways) and inhibition of erythrocyte cholinesterase activity.

In the early 1950s, Dr David Grob (then associated with The Johns Hopkins Hospital) and associates investigated the clinical pharmacology of sarin in an elaborate series of studies extending over several years. They administered the agent orally, intra-arterially, percutaneously and topically in the eye, and described the clinical and laboratory effects, including those on the electroencephalogram. They noted that the erythrocyte cholinesterase activity was inhibited to a greater degree than the plasma enzyme, but that the plasma enzyme recovered faster. They also noted that atropine was effective at reversing the effects in organs with muscarinic receptor sites. They published their studies in numerous government contract reports. Since these findings are also published in journals that are readily available,[10-12] they will not be detailed here. Over the several-year duration of these studies, the secrecy surrounding the compounds decreased. In the first report[10] the investigators described the effects of 'nerve gas', but the agent is not mentioned nor are doses given. Later, both the specific agent and the doses were included. These reports contain the familiar table showing the effects of nerve agents that has been reproduced in many places, including military manuals.

Skin exposure

The toxicity of liquid nerve agents on the skin was studied extensively. In the first study reported,[13] 5-mg droplets of sarin (6–129 droplets; total doses of 25–550 mg) were placed on the volar aspects of the forearms of 11 subjects. The agent evaporated in 1.5–6 min from the skin when the area was relatively free of hair, and in 6.5–15 min from the skin when placed in areas of heavy hair. The agent was mixed with a dye for visualization, and after evaporation was complete the site was tested for the agent and then decontaminated. Maximal inhibition of erythrocyte cholinesterase activity was 18% (82% of normal). Two subjects (cholinesterase of 82%) had transient diarrhea. Sweating at the site of application continued for as long as 34 days.

A small amount (3.21 mg) of liquid sarin was applied to the skin of six subjects, and about 98% of it was recovered in the air.[14] The tendency of sarin to evaporate rather than to penetrate skin was noted in a later, more extensive study.[15] In a similar study by two of the same investigators,[16] tabun, 50–400 mg in 0.5-mg droplets was placed on the volar aspects of forearm skin of six subjects. The droplets evaporated in 18–167 min, and the maximal inhibition of erythrocyte cholinesterase activity was 34% (in a subject who received 400 μg kg^{-1}). Sweating, a feeling of coolness and blanching occurred at the site after exposure, and localized sweating persisted for 8–95 days. Ambient temperatures were about 24°C, relative humidities about 40%, and wind speed about 1 mile per hour in these two studies.

In an extensive study,[15] sarin in amounts of 30–300 mg as 0.5-mg droplets was placed on the bare forearm skin of 114 subjects at a temperature of 70°F (21°C) and a relative humidity of 70%. In contrast to the studies noted above, in which decontamination was not done until the droplet had been absorbed or had evaporated, the site of application was decontaminated 30 min after exposure. The average inhibition of erythrocyte cholinesterase at the highest dose was 40%, but the variation was large. Four subjects had inhibition of greater than 80%; three of these had no effects and one had generalized sweating with cold clammy skin and vomiting, and was given atropine. Amounts of 100–300 mg (0.5-mg droplets) of sarin were placed on one layer of serge over the forearm skin. The mean inhibition of cholinesterase activity at the highest dose was 48%. Four subjects, each with more than 85% inhibition of erythrocyte cholinesterase, vomited starting 30 min to 26 h after exposure. A fifth had profuse sweating and difficulty in breathing soon after decontamination and were treated with antibiotics. Sarin, 200 mg (0.5-mg droplets), was placed on a layer of serge over a layer of flannel on the forearm skin of 18 subjects. Mean erythrocyte cholinesterase inhibition was 43% (this amount had caused 25% inhibition when placed on serge and 19% on bare skin). One subject with 96% inhibition of erythrocyte cholinesterase had generalized muscular fasciculations and difficulty in respiration 23 min after the start of exposure and was treated. No subject with less than 80% inhibition in erythrocyte cholinesterase activity had any effects from the agent.

In another part of this study, soman, 10–40 mg in 0.5-mg droplets, was placed on the forearms of 32 subjects. The mean erythrocyte cholinesterase inhibition increased from 13% to 27% as the dose increased. GF (another organophosphorus cholinesterase inhibitor and nerve agent), in doses of 5–30 mg in 0.5-mg droplets, produced a mean inhibition of 57% after the highest amount. Several doses of soman and GF, given as single drops, caused 2–10 times more inhibition of cholinesterase than when given as multiple small droplets. The time course of cholinesterase inhibition was not detailed. The amounts of agent needed to inhibit erythrocyte cholinesterase activity by 50% when placed on bare skin were estimated to be 400 mg per person for sarin, 65 mg per person for soman, and 30 mg per person for GF.

In a later study,[17] 0.2–6.1 mg of soman was placed on the forearms of subjects in an open ward. Several subjects and the investigators had eye effects from agent vapor, but there were no systemic effects or inhibition of erythrocyte cholinesterase. The next part of this study took place in a static chamber, with the investigators watching through a window, where 2.0–7.8 mg was applied to the forearm skin of 25 subjects. Most had localized sweating at the site of application. On several days of the study when the ambient temperature was over 80°F (27°C) and relative humidity over 85%, the cholinesterase activity inhibition was slightly greater than on the other days when temperature and humidity were lower. Otherwise, maximal inhibition of erythrocyte cholinesterase activity occurred between 2 and 24 h after exposure, and the maximal inhibition was to 69% of baseline.

Exposure of skin to vapor

One arm of each of four subjects was put into a chamber and exposed to Cts of 1000–8000 mg min m^{-3} of tabun.[18] There were no effects or changes in plasma cholinesterase activity. Later, 16 subjects dressed in shoes, shorts and protective masks were exposed to Cts of 520–2000 mg min m^{-3} of tabun (roughly 5–10 times the estimated LCt_{50} of tabun by inhalation). The cholinesterase activity was inhibited more at 1 h after exposure than at 15 min after exposure, but at neither time was it markedly inhibited. There was a slight but statistically significant difference between the cholinesterase activity of the group exposed to 520–970 mg min m^{-3} (between 90% and 100% of control) and that of the group exposed to 1320–2000 mg min m^{-3} (80–90%). There were no signs or symptoms, and electrocardiograms and blood pressures were normal. In a similar study, effects were minimal after skin exposure to about 10–15 times the inhalational LCt_{50} of sarin.

Performance studies

The potential effects of nerve agents on intellectual, cognitive or psychomotor functioning were examined in several studies. Sarin was the agent in each study. Twenty subjects who received a Ct of 10 mg min m^{-3} had no deterioration in central intellectual capacity, but were impaired slightly on a visual search task, and their rate of learning on a hand–eye task was slower 5 and 24 h after exposure than before exposure. Extra stress caused their performance to deteriorate further, and they were noted to be lethargic and disinclined to be bothered.[19]

In a similar study by the same investigator,[20] 12 subjects received a Ct of 14.7 mg min m^{-3}, and 12 non-exposed subjects were controls. Again, intellectual capacity was not impaired. However, the perceptual span was slightly less and the flicker threshold frequency (FTF) was decreased in the exposed subjects. Their three-dimensional space coordination was markedly impaired. The decrease in FTF was similar to that seen with fatigue.

In a third study,[21] eight subjects received a Ct of 14.6 mg min m^{-3} (which inhibited their erythrocyte cholinesterase activity by an average of 36%). At 5 and 24 h after exposure, there was no serious intellectual decline, but cognitive function was slightly decreased and subjects had a decrease in manual dexterity/discrimination, possibly because of finger incoordination. Self-rating scales indicated that the subjects had dysphoria and reduced mental alertness.

Twenty-eight subjects who received a rather low Ct of 4 mg min m^{-3} with 17% inhibition of erythrocyte cholinesterase activity took a battery of tests, including the Minnesota rate of manipulation, Purdue pegboard, dual pursuit meter, reaction time, a steadiness aiming device, and an addition task.[22] Although their pupil sizes had decreased by at least 2 mm, their performance was not severely impaired on any task and was improved on many.

No changes in performance were found on a heavy pursuit meter task, a light pursuit meter task, and a ball bearing picking task in 25 subjects who received 5 μg kg^{-1} of vapor by oral inhalation (eyes not exposed).[23]

Intellectual function was examined in 24 individuals who had been accidentally exposed to sarin.[24] They were divided into high- and low-dose groups based on their clinical signs and the judgement of the investigators. Subscales of the Wechsler–Bellevue test were used. The only differences between immediate post-exposure tests and baseline tests (tests done several months after exposure when the individuals were considered to have completely recovered) were on the similarities and comprehension scales in the high-dose group. These differences appeared to indicate impairment of judgement and of higher-level verbal concept formation.

A study of behavioral changes in humans after VX is noted in the section on VX.

Physical performance

Several studies examined physical performance after sarin. In the first,[25] two groups of 20 subjects each received 5 μg kg^{-1} of sarin using the single-breath technique of oral inhalation. (In the single-breath technique the subject breathed a measured amount of air containing a known amount of agent through a mouthpiece with nose clamped and with no eye exposure. The amount is given as μg kg^{-1}. When the amount is given as a Ct, the subject generally was exposed in a chamber with no protection to eyes, nose or mouth. The exact inhaled dose is not known with the latter method.) Because of vapor condensation on the apparatus, the first group did not receive the full amount of sarin, and their mean erythrocyte cholinesterase activity was depressed by only 18%. They rode a bicycle ergometer as fast as possible for 5 min per day for 5 days and inhaled the sarin just before the ride on day 3. The incidence of chest symptoms was lower than usual during the ride, and some felt the ride was easier than usual. Some complained of a tight chest 10–15 min after the ride. There were no changes in minute volume, oxygen intake, or carbon dioxide output. Another group rode the bicycle at a constant rate for 15 min three times a day for 10 days and inhaled sarin on day 8 (mean erythrocyte cholinesterase activity was 65% of baseline). There was a small but insignificant increase in oxygen consumption but no other changes.

In a later study,[26] 14 subjects exposed to a Ct of 14.7 mg min m^{-3} of sarin (mean erythrocyte inhibition of 50%) carried one-third of their body weight up and down a

40.5-cm step 30 times a minute for 5 min (the Harvard pack test). This was done 45 min and 24 h after exposure. Their fitness index, which includes heart rate and other measures, did not differ from that of a group exposed to agent but not exercised.

Physiology

Needle electrodes were placed in intercostal muscles in 10 subjects who received 70–150 μg of sarin by the single-breath technique of vapor administration.[27] Although eight noted chest tightness, none had changes in whole blood cholinesterase, and there were no abnormalities in the electrical pattern from the muscles. It was concluded that muscular abnormalities did not contribute to the sensation of dyspnea.

Venous tone in the legs was examined by a g-suit technique in 23 subjects who received 5 μg kg^{-1} of sarin by the single-breath technique of vapor exposure (33% decrease in erythrocyte cholinesterase activity).[28] Although there was a small decrease in the average tidal volume and a small increase in the respiratory rate in these subjects, there was no change in the amount of end-tidal shift of air in the lungs (which would have suggested a change in venous return). This suggested that pressor amines probably would not be useful in therapy of sarin intoxication.

Using a low-frequency critically damped ballistocardiograph, cardiac output was estimated in 25 subjects given 5 μg kg^{-1} of sarin by oral inhalation (which caused a mean 37% decrease in erythrocyte cholinesterase activity). There was a small increase in heart rate, which the investigator felt was a cortical response to the sensation of a tight chest, but no changes in cardiac output were noted.[29]

Fifteen subjects were simultaneously acclimatized to heat and cold by spending part of each day in a hot chamber and part in a cold chamber.[30] After acclimatization had been achieved (as determined by appropriate techniques), eight of the subjects received sarin by inhalation (a Ct of 15 mg min m^{-3}). Physiological studies indicated they did not differ from the unexposed acclimatized group, and it was concluded that the agent did not interfere with acclimatization.

Odor

At a concentration of sarin under 1.5 mg m^{-3}, 8 of 15 people noted an odor, but gave no good description of it and did not think that they would recognize it again.[31] In contrast, 14 of 15 described a stronger musty, spicy or fruity odor after sniffing a similar concentration of soman and thought that they would recognize it again.

About 50% of 34 subjects (22 male and 12 female laboratory workers) detected the odor of soman in concentrations of 3.3–7.0 mg m^{-3} and described it as sweet, fruity or nutty.[32] About 65% of the subjects had mild nasal and airway symptoms from the agent.

Twenty people were exposed to GF vapor. At a concentration of 10.4 mg m^{-3}, 35% could smell it, and 65% could detect an odor at a concentration of 14.8 mg m^{-3}.[33] There was no agreement on the odor.

Miscellaneous

Dressed subjects wearing the standard US M17 mask, hood and combat uniform (not protective clothing) were exposed for 20 min to concentrations of sarin of 0.25–4.8 mg m^{-3} or for 5 min at concentrations of 8.9–27.1 mg m^{-3}. (Absorption through the skin is negligible under these circumstances.) While in the vapor atmosphere, they carefully removed their mask and hood to eat or drink. They could take a bite or a sip of liquid in an average of 4 s, and the total unprotected time while they ate rations or drank some water ranged from 0.21 to 1.5 min. Many had miosis and rhinorrhea and complained of chest tightness. The inhibition of whole blood cholinesterase activity ranged from 2% to 32%. Those who only drank expired deeply before removing their mask, effectively clearing it, had no symptoms or physical signs, and averaged 26% inhibition of cholinesterase activity. The investigator concluded that it was safe to eat and drink in a contaminated atmosphere if these activities are done carefully.[34]

Pulmonary

In a study using 150 laboratory employees and enlisted personnel, pulmonary function (vital capacity and maximum breathing capacity) was examined after various Cts to 6.0 mg min m^{-3}.[35] There was a good correlation between degree of bronchoconstriction and Ct over the dose range used (0.7). Maximal bronchoconstriction occurred between 15 min and 2 h after exposure, with a tendency to recover by 3 h. Although subjects were directed to breathe through their noses only, one also breathed through his mouth and had more severe symptoms and pulmonary function decrement. This suggested that nasal breathing offers some protection.

Using the same 150 subjects at the same time, another investigator measured airway resistance with an interrupted-flow technique. He found minimal airway obstruction and that only at the highest Ct.[36]

In another study, 105 subjects inhaled Cts ranging from 2.4 to 19.6 mg min m^{-3} (retained doses of 0.1–3.1 μg kg^{-1}). There was a mean erythrocyte cholinesterase inhibition of 30% at a retained dose of 2.2 μg kg^{-1} and a 'rough' correlation of enzyme inhibition with retained dose. However, although measures of pulmonary function varied widely both above and below baseline, none changed consistently with dose. Measures used included resting tidal volume, exercise tidal volume, maximum breathing capacity, and vital capacity.[37]

Using a single-breath technique of sarin administration, 63 subjects inhaled doses of 0.6–3.3 μg kg^{-1}. Increase in airway resistance was dose dependent, but it correlated better with the concentration of agent (which varied from 5 to 40 mg m^{-3}) than with Ct. At the highest dose, resistance was 2.9 times baseline at 1 min after exposure, 2 times baseline at 15 min, and 1.6 times baseline at 1 h. At lower amounts, resistance was less and improvement was faster. The incidence and severity of airway symptoms paralleled the time course of the increased resistance.

Symptoms were maximal immediately after exposure and improved over the next 15 min.[38]

Also with a single-breath technique, 25 subjects inhaled 0.5–5.0 μg kg^{-1} of sarin and had fewer symptoms than usually seen after these amounts.[39] There was a correlation between the amount retained and erythrocyte cholinesterase inhibition, with a maximal inhibition of 27% at 5.0 μg kg^{-1}. The half-time for inhibition of the enzyme was about 90 s, and inhibition was complete in about 10 min.

The same investigator[40] administered a dose of 0.5 μg kg^{-1} on two occasions to four subjects and a dose of 2.5 μg kg^{-1} on two occasions to 29 others. In each group, the rate of inhalation varied with each exposure. Symptoms depended on the rate of inhalation. A flow rate of 20 l min^{-1} caused a minimal change in pulmonary resistance, and symptoms were related to the tongue and throat as well as chest. At a rate over 40 l min^{-1}, there was a marked increase in pulmonary resistance, and symptoms were confined to the chest. The investigator suggested that at lower rates much of the vapor is absorbed in the upper airways and that at higher rates absorption is primarily in the lower airways. Erythrocyte cholinesterase activity inhibition was 17–20% in both groups.

Others studied the absorption of sarin vapor in rabbits, monkeys and humans.[41,42] Retention in the nasal tract and trachea was 98% in rabbits and 93% in monkeys, leaving little to be absorbed in the terminal airways. During nasal breathing humans retained 96% of inhaled sarin.

In the first of two related studies by the same investigators,[43,44] subjects retained 82% of orally inhaled sarin while at rest and 81% while exercising on a bicycle ergometer. In the second study, 52 subjects breathing orally retained 87% of inhaled sarin and 39 subjects breathing nasally retained 89% of the agent. When exposed to sarin vapor while exercising and breathing orally, 41 subjects retained 80%. The estimated retained amounts to reduce the erythrocyte cholinesterase activity by 50% were 3.73 μg kg^{-1} for oral inhalation at rest, 4.06 μg kg^{-1} for nasal inhalation at rest, and 4.43 μg kg^{-1} for oral inhalation while exercising. The investigators remarked that because the minute volume was about eight times greater in the exercising subjects, the concentration was decreased by a factor of about eight, and that minute volume must be considered when using the term Ct.[45,46]

Using a mathematical model and data from other sources (not stated, but probably from the above studies), an investigator suggested that after oral inhalation of sarin at low flow rates about 50–70% is absorbed in the upper airway and 20–40% in the lungs (lower airways), while about 20% is exhaled. At high flow rates, these are essentially reversed, with about 20% absorption in the upper airway, 50–70% in the lungs (lower airways), and 10–30% exhaled.[47]

Military effectiveness

One of the first studies done with a nerve agent in humans concerned soldiers' abilities to conduct military operations after exposure to the agent.[5] A similar study was done with 134 enlisted soldiers and five officers exposed to sarin at Cts of 11.8–

13.9 mg min m^{-3}.[48] After exposure, all subjects had miosis, about 75% had rhinorrhea (which decreased by 5 h), about half complained of a headache, and fewer than half noted the sensation of a tight chest. They conducted an approach march, an attack with support weapons, controlled firing, and a twilight advance into position. In addition, night patrols were sent on a compass route. The conclusions included the comments that the men showed more signs of fatigue than normal, that commanders became irritable and unduly flustered, and that accuracy and speed of lower ranks were not up to normal. The investigators felt that most normal military operations could be conducted satisfactorily except for those at night.

In a similar exercise, 169 subjects received Cts of about 12 mg min m^{-3} and then were divided into four groups.[49] Signs and symptoms were the same as had been noted in previous studies: eye effects, rhinorrhea and dyspnea. One group then received atropine, one group wore respirators after exposure, one group received atropine and wore respirators, and one group received neither atropine nor respirators after exposure. The conclusions suggested that after exposure to agent and administration of atropine, operations may be hazardous by day and would definitely be dangerous by night because of impaired eyesight and mental alertness. Masking after exposure increased the basic mental harassment and produced distress during intense physical effort. With the combination of masking and atropine, the deleterious effects were additive.

Eye

The first studies on these agents focused on eye effects,[4,5] and many later ones concentrated on this organ. In subjects exposed to Cts of 1 to 6 mg min m^{-3}, a linear relationship was noted between Ct and decrease in pupil size. At a Ct of 1 mg min m^{-3} the decrease was 1.1 mm, and at a Ct of 6 mg min m^{-3} the decrease was 3.0 mm. Near and far points did not change.[50]

Of a total of 240 subjects, one group had their eyes 'bandaged' (not complete occlusion), other groups had no protection, and another group received 2 mg of atropine intramuscularly 0.5 h before all were exposed to Cts of 5–15 mg min m^{-3} of sarin.[51] The Ct of 5 mg min m^{-3} caused slower and less complete constriction than the higher Cts. Bandaged eyes constricted more slowly and less completely. Although atropine decreased conjunctival suffusion and complaints of eye pain, it appeared not to affect the miosis.

The sensitivity of human and rabbit eyes to agents was compared in a study in which the agent was administered in air flowing through tightly fitting goggles (in both the humans and the rabbits).[52] By this technique, the ECt$_{50}$ (Ct to produce the effect in 50% of the population) for miosis after sarin was 3.13 mg min m^{-3} for humans and 2.33 mg min m^{-3} for the animals. At a concentration of 3.7 mg m^{-3} there was a delay of several minutes for miosis after sarin and soman, but a delay of 30–40 min after VX. The ECts to cause miosis in the rabbit in a static chamber were 1.32 mg min m^{-3} for sarin, 0.59 mg min m^{-3} for soman, and 0.04 mg min m^{-3} for VX. The investigators commented that VX might cause miosis in concentrations under the limits of field detectors. These data also illustrate the reason that rabbits were felt to be very effective detectors of agent.

Various measures of eye function were examined in 27 volunteers who received Cts of 1.87–15 mg min m^{-3} of sarin.[53] Miosis was maximal within 30 min in all except the lowest dose group. The contrast threshold changed by 23% at the highest Ct and by 15% in the next highest dose group and correlated well with the square of the pupillary diameter. There was no change in visual acuity and little (under 1D) change in refractive state. The near point decreased. The symptoms included pain on convergence with an increase in pain with increased illumination. The conclusion was that an aircrew would function well in daytime even at the highest Ct (15 mg min m^{-3}), but that at night the maximal allowable Ct should be 2 mg min m^{-3}.

Six subjects were exposed to a Ct of 15 mg min m^{-3} of sarin vapor.[54] Visual acuity was unchanged after the exposure (it was actually improved in one subject), despite the subjects' complaints to the contrary. The topical instillation of cyclopentolate markedly decreased near visual ability. The investigators suggested that topical mydriatics be reserved for those needing night vision or those with marked discomfort from the eye changes.

In a series of studies,[55–58] Rubin and associates investigated the effects of sarin on night vision. Inhalation of sarin (in a chamber) with full eye protection caused an elevation of the scotopic threshold (decreased ability to perceive light in darkness) even though miosis was not present. Local instillation of sarin into an eye caused miosis, but not an increase in the scotopic threshold. When one eye was completely protected (miosis did not occur) and the other exposed to sarin vapor which the subject inhaled, the protected eye did not become miotic but there was an increased threshold in both eyes. Finally, after sarin exposure intramuscular administration of atropine sulfate (which enters the central nervous system) reversed the increased threshold, whereas injection of atropine methylnitrate (which does not enter the central nervous system) did not. The investigators concluded that the decreased ability to perceive light is related to central mechanisms, possibly in the retina or visual pathways, rather than to miosis.

In another study,[59,60] miosis was induced by inhalation of sarin or by physostigmine eye drops. Although the degree of miosis was equal, the subjects with sarin exposure were less able to perceive a stimulus of standard luminance. This study concluded, as had the previously described study, that effects on central pathways rather than miosis *per se* were the primary determinants of the agent-induced visual deficit.

However, the amount of elevation of the scotopic threshold did correlate with decrease in pupillary area in 10 subjects who received sarin eye drops.[61] The investigators in this study concluded that the decrease in night vision was directly related to miosis alone.

In three workers accidentally exposed to sarin, the return of the ability of the iris to dilate correlated better with return of plasma cholinesterase activity than with return of erythrocyte enzyme activity.[62] The dark-adapted pupil size, measured in complete darkness, did not return to normal for about 6 weeks.

Two other workers accidentally exposed also exhibited slow recovery of pupillary function.[63] Visual acuity was temporarily improved by sarin in these presbyopic subjects.

Studies with protection

The oxime 2-pralidoxime chloride (2-PAMCl) was administered by slow intravenous infusion to subjects who had received sarin. The half-time for *in vivo* aging of the sarin–erythrocyte complex seemed to be about 5 h.[64]

Sarin was given intravenously to counteract the effects of intoxication by a cholinergic blocking compound in two subjects.[65] It caused total inhibition of erythrocyte cholinesterase activity in one subject and reversed both the central nervous system and more peripherally mediated effects of the anticholinergic compound in both subjects. There were no effects from sarin.

VX

Intravenous

Human studies with VX began in 1959 when an investigator, Dr Van M. Sim, volunteered to be the first subject. VX, 0.04 μg kg^{-1}, was given intravenously over 30 s with no untoward effects and no change in erythrocyte cholinesterase activity. Three and a half hours later, 0.08 μg kg^{-1} was administered by the same method. He developed a headache, felt sweaty and lightheaded, and complained of abdominal cramps, but blood cholinesterase activity was normal. For regulatory and approval reasons, a year intervened before the study continued.

Again, Dr Sim was the initial subject and received a 30-s injection of 0.225 μg kg^{-1} of VX which caused a decrease in erythrocyte cholinesterase activity to 63% of baseline. After 2 h, an intravenous infusion of 1 μg min^{-1} was begun. A variety of minor effects occurred during the infusion, but at 3.5 h he became pale, stopped talking, appeared 'out of contact', and had profuse salivation and vomiting. The confusional state lasted about 15 min. It was learned later that his erythrocyte cholinesterase activity was 15% of his baseline.[66]

In a continuation of this study, six other subjects received 1 μg kg^{-1} of VX by slow intravenous infusion. Their average erythrocyte cholinesterase activity ranged from 34% to 45% of their control activities.

In a later study, 27 subjects received 1.3–1.5 μg kg^{-1} of VX intravenously over 30 s.[67] By 15 min, 12 subjects (with erythrocyte cholinesterase activities 17–45% of controls) were dizzy, shaky or lightheaded. Of 17 subjects who later had erythrocyte cholinesterase activity of less than 30% of their baseline, five vomited and two were treated for severe nausea. Of eight with enzyme activity less than 25%, four vomited, two were treated for severe nausea, and one complained of nausea. These severe effects occurred more than an hour after agent administration. The time of maximal inhibition of erythrocyte cholinesterase activity was also about an hour after agent administration. Recovery of the enzyme was about 1% per hour for the first day or two.

VX was also administered intravenously as an antidote for intoxication with cholinergic blocking compounds.[68] It was extremely effective at reversing both the central and peripheral effects of these compounds. There were no other effects from the agent.

Vapor exposure

The forearm or the entire arm of 29 subjects was exposed to *Ct*s of 7–681 mg min m^{-3} of VX vapor.[69] Blood was taken for whole blood cholinesterase activity once before exposure and once at 20 h after exposure. (Because the VX-inhibited cholinesterase reactivates rapidly during the first hours after inhibition, this may not be a good measure of the maximal amount of inhibition.) The enzyme activity was inhibited in a dose-related fashion from 3% to 43%. There were neither signs nor symptoms.

The heads and necks of medical officers were exposed to VX vapor on 54 occasions.[70] (Because the VX-inhibited cholinesterase recovers rapidly, the same few subjects were used repeatedly.) On 19 occasions there was no respiratory protection (*Ct*s of 0.6 mg min m^{-3} to 6.4 mg min m^{-3}), and on 35 occasions the respiratory tract was protected by having the subjects breathe clean air through a tube with the nose clamped (*Ct*s of 0.7 mg min m^{-3} to 25.6 mg min m^{-3}). In the unprotected subjects, some had miosis even though their eyes had been closed; the onset of miosis was about 1–3 h after exposure (and possibly could have been from vapor from the skin exposure). Chest tightness and rhinorrhea occurred from 7 min to 30 min after exposure. There was no significant inhibition in erythrocyte cholinesterase activity immediately after exposure, but there was some inhibition at 15 min after exposure, and maximal inhibition occurred at 4 h. Most of the subjects who were exposed only by skin exposure had miosis within 0.5–4 h after exposure, and two also had nausea. The erythrocyte cholinesterase activity did not change within the first 20 min, and maximal inhibition occurred at 8–12 h. The investigators noted the slower onset of effects from VX vapor compared to sarin vapor (onset of effects is slow even after intravenous administration of VX[67]).

The recovery of VX-inhibited erythrocyte cholinesterase activity was studied after the enzyme had been inhibited by percutaneous or inhalational exposure (in other studies).[71] The enzyme recovered at a rate of 6% per day for the first 3–4 days, and then at 1% per day. A rapid early recovery of the enzyme was noted in several other studies.

Application on the skin

VX, in amounts of 5–35 μg kg^{-1} in small droplets, was applied to the volar aspect of the forearms of 103 subjects. The ambient temperature was 70–80°F and the relative humidity ranged from 40% to 70%.[72] Under these conditions, the amount estimated to produce a 50% inhibition of erythrocyte cholinesterase activity was 34 μg kg^{-1}. Symptoms, which usually occurred later than 6 h after exposure, included local sweating at the site (local muscular fasciculations were seen in only two subjects), a feeling of tiredness or weakness, nausea, vomiting, and headaches. The incidence of vomiting was related to inhibition of cholinesterase; after more than 70–80% inhibition of erythrocyte cholinesterase activity, more than half of the subjects vomited. There were few symptoms when cholinesterase activity was about 50% of normal, but symptoms increased in severity and duration as the enzyme activity fell below 30% of baseline activity. When VX was mixed with an amine (1 : 1), absorption of the agent was enhanced.

Amounts of VX of 5–30 μg kg^{-1} were applied to 19 different skin sites in a large group of subjects.[73] The estimated amount to cause a 70% reduction in erythrocyte cholinesterase activity varied by a factor of 26, from 5.1 μg kg^{-1} on the cheek to 132 μg kg^{-1} on the palm. The ear (6.6 μg kg^{-1}), top of the head (10.8 μg kg^{-1}), and forehead (11.2 μg kg^{-1}) were among the more sensitive areas of skin, while the dorsal forearm (93.8 μg kg^{-1}), dorsal foot (94.3 μg kg^{-1}) and knee (102 μg kg^{-1}) were among the least sensitive. Thirty-two subjects had a maximal drop in erythrocyte cholinesterase activity of 70% or more, and 25 of these became sick. The median time of onset of illness was 5 h after application of the agent to the head, 7 h for the extremities, and 10 h for the trunk. When the agent was applied to bearded skin, both the amount of inhibition of cholinesterase and the symptoms were more severe. The oximes 2-PAMCl and P2S reactivated the inhibited cholinesterase and reduced the severity of the symptoms.

Radiolabeled (^{32}P) VX was applied to the palm (26 μg), the back (25 μg) or the forearm (15.7 μg) of several subjects, and the amount in the skin and the amount recovered by washing the site were counted.[74] Based on a decrease of whole blood cholinesterase activity of 3%, the investigators concluded that less than 1% had penetrated through the palm skin, 8% the skin of the back, and 15% the skin of the forearm.

Neat VX, 20 μg kg^{-1}, was applied to the skin of four subjects, while four other subjects received 20 μg kg^{-1} mixed 1 : 1 with octylamine, and four others received neat VX, 35 μg kg^{-1}.[75] Seven were symptomatic with insomnia, nightmares, lightheadedness, nausea, epigastric discomfort, vomiting and diarrhea. (The whole blood activity was 14–38% of control in these subjects.) The whole blood erythrocyte activity was above 42% of control activity in the five asymptomatic subjects. Plasma and urinary electrolytes, BSP excretion, SGOT, SGPT and serum amylase were all normal following exposure.

One subject received neat VX on one occasion and VX mixed with n-octylamine on another (3 : 1, amine/VX).[76] Absorption of agent was increased by the amine (maximal erythrocyte cholinesterase activity inhibition of 9% with agent alone, and 41% with the mixture).

In two large and elaborate studies, Craig, Cummings and associates studied the penetration of VX through the skin of the cheek and forearm at ambient temperatures of 0°F, 35°F, 65°F and 115°F.[77,78] Because these studies are reported elsewhere[79] they will not be described in detail. Among their conclusions were that absorption of agent was faster and more complete at higher temperatures (27% more per 10°F increase in temperature) and that absorption continued for hours after decontamination of the application site (usually with 5.25% hypochlorite). The onset of effects and maximal inhibition of erythrocyte cholinesterase activity typically occurred several hours after the conclusion of the 3-h exposure (at which time the site was decontaminated).

The arms of three medical officers were covered with an outer layer of battledress serge over flannel and 200 mg of VX (as droplets of 0.8–1.61 μl) was dropped on the serge and allowed to remain for 8 h.[80] (The current estimate for the LD_{50} for VX liquid on the skin is 10 mg.) About 85% of the agent was recovered from the serge and about 5% from the flannel. The investigators suggested that the remainder evaporated. The subjects had no symptoms and no decrease in erythrocyte cholinesterase activity.

Later, under the same experimental conditions VX was allowed to remain on the serge in two subjects for 24 h. Erythrocyte cholinesterase activity began to fall within 14 h, and at 24 h, when the material was removed and the arms decontaminated (5.25% hypochlorite), it was 73% in one subject and 81% in the other. Maximal inhibition of the enzyme (34% and 64% of baseline) occurred at 48 h and 24 h after decontamination. The activity of the lower cholinesterase returned at a rate of about 10% per day for the next 3 days, but then slowed to about 1% per day. Both subjects were symptom- and sign-free. (This study should be compared to that in which sarin was placed on serge and flannel and left in place for 30 min.)

Ingestion

Fifty-four subjects drank water contaminated with VX to find the time to incipient toxicity, defined as inhibition of erythrocyte cholinesterase activity of 70% or more.[81] Doses of VX and types of water were varied. At an amount of 400 μg per 70 kg in distilled water, cholinesterase activity fell to 22% of the control activity in 1 day. With the same amount in distilled water to which tetraglycine hydroperiodide (a water-purifying agent) was added, the mean cholinesterase activity was 17% of control activity in 16 h. At the same dose in water treated with the standard field kit for chemical agent decontamination of water, toxicity occurred on day 4 in four of eight subjects. The same amount of VX added to tap water produced toxicity in six of nine subjects on day 4 also. Doses of 100–125 mg per 70 kg caused incipient toxicity in 6–7 days.

Maximal cholinesterase inhibition occurred in 2–3 h in subjects who drank VX in saline or dextrose in water.[82] At the same doses, eating before ingesting VX enhanced absorption. When the agent was mixed with tap water instead of with saline or dextrose in water, absorption was less. About 2.5 μg kg^{-1} of VX caused a

50% inhibition of erythrocyte cholinesterase activity, and 3.8 μg kg^{-1} produced a 70% inhibition.

When given orally, VX was ineffective in reversing the intoxication caused by a cholinergic blocking component, even though an equipotent amount (the amount causing the same inhibition of erythrocyte cholinesterase activity) given intravenously produced very effective antagonism.[68]

Psychological effects

Psychological and behavioral effects were studied in 93 subjects who had been exposed to VX on the skin.[83] (Results from skin exposure were reported in references 72 and 73; in this report the agent is referred to as EA 1701.) About 30% of subjects had symptoms of anxiety, 57% had psychomotor depression and 57% had intellectual impairment after inhibition of whole blood cholinesterase activity by more than 60% (or below 40% of their baseline activity). (As the erythrocyte cholinesterase activity is usually about half that of the whole blood after VX exposure, this suggests that these subjects had about 20% of their control erythrocyte cholinesterase activity.) Fewer than 10% of the subjects with less enzyme inhibition had these effects. Psychological effects usually appeared earlier than physical effects (nausea, vomiting) or appeared in the absence of physical effects. The psychological effects were characterized by difficulty in sustaining attention and a slowing of intellectual and motor processes. There were no illogical or inappropriate trends in language and thinking, no conceptual looseness, and no perceptual distortions.

Odor

Half of a group of subjects smelled VX at a concentration of 3.9 mg m^{-3}. When two different stabilizers were added, the odor was detectable at 1.9 and 1.0 mg m^{-3}. However, the odor was not clearly described.[84]

Therapeutic studies

Subjects given VX in other studies received the oxime 2-PAMCl (by slow intravenous infusion) at times as long as 48 h after VX administration. Significant reactivation of the inhibited erythrocyte cholinesterase activity occurred at all times, even though the doses of oxime were small (5–25 mg kg^{-1}). Aging of the VX–enzyme complex occurs later than 48 h or possibly not at all.[64]

An experimental VX-like compound was given intravenously to 30 subjects.[85] The dose to cause 70% inhibition of erythrocyte cholinesterase activity was estimated to be 0.99 μg kg^{-1}. Four subjects had symptoms of lightheadedness, anorexia, fatigue, and difficulty in sleeping. More severe effects did not occur, although three subjects had erythrocyte cholinesterase activity less than 10% of their baselines. 2-PAMCl, given 3 min after agent administration, did not affect the enzyme activity.

ACCIDENTAL EXPOSURES

During the research, developmental and manufacturing programs there were many accidental exposures to these agents. Almost all were vapor exposures to sarin. Most were considered mild, and few casualties were given therapy. At the height of the program, the sudden onset of 'dim vision', a runny nose and tightness in the chest was not considered the serious matter that it might be today. Individuals have told the author that they continued work under these circumstances rather than seek medical attention. (This occurred despite emphasis by management and medical staff on prompt reporting of even minor symptoms.)

The large majority of reported instances of accidental exposure had one or more of these effects. Very often there was associated pain in the head, a vague sensation of 'not feeling well', nausea, and perhaps some very mild intellectual or cognitive slowing. Sometimes there were no objective signs of exposure, but only complaints of dyspnea, nausea, or 'not feeling well'. In the earlier years this was compounded by lack of cholinesterase monitoring, so this evidence was absent also. Several years ago the author reviewed the records of the medical facility at Edgewood Arsenal dating from the late 1940s. About 200 records had objective evidence of exposure noted on the medical chart (miosis, depressed cholinesterase activity, rhinorrhea, obvious signs of respiratory difficulty), although many times that number of records did not report any objective evidence even though the patient had reported to the facility because of nerve agent exposure. A report published in a medical journal in 1959 described 22 typical cases.[86]

Four severe exposures have been reported. They will be discussed later.

The largest number of exposures reported at a single facility were those discussed in two separate reports from Rocky Mountain Arsenal.[87,88] Each report tabulates over 300 exposures, but some cases may have been listed in both. Fewer than 4% of the patients were treated, and of those who were treated, some were in a study of whether orally administered atropine or a placebo provided the better therapy. (Atropine appeared to provide more relief in the more severe cases, but in the mild exposures there was no difference between the two.)

Two investigators reported effects in themselves from accidental exposure.[89,90] The first report described an investigator and some of his staff who were exposed to soman vapor with ensuing miosis, headache, general malaise, and some impairment of intellectual abilities. The second report documents more severe effects. The investigator had serious breathing difficulties and severe muscular spasms, but did not lose consciousness, convulse, or stop breathing. He received large amounts of atropine (45 mg within the first hour) and experienced mental difficulties, including inability to concentrate for weeks afterwards. Although the time of their return varied, all of these scientists resumed their normal work.

The earliest report of accidental exposures described 10 cases.[91] Over the next decade other reports described about 200 cases of exposure to G agents[92-97] and about 20 cases of exposure to VX-like agents (although none to VX).[98,99]

The first severe exposure was described in 1952.[100,101] A physician was suddenly exposed to a large concentration of sarin. Within seconds he lost consciousness and convulsed. A minute or two later he became apneic. The second case was a subject in an experimental program who had a more severe toxic effect from a small amount of sarin on his abraded skin than others had had.[12] A third individual had a small leak in his protective mask while working in an atmosphere of sarin.[62] He exited the area, suddenly lost consciousness, convulsed, and became apneic. A chemist was pipetting a solution containing soman and got some in and around his mouth.[62] He went to the medical facility, where he lost consciousness in about 15 min after the exposure. Medical assistance was available almost immediately for all four of these individuals, and all survived. Cases one (a physician), three (a technician) and four (a chemist) resumed their normal work after 6–8 weeks with no known decrements. The further effects, if any, in case two were not reported.

CONCLUSION

Over a two-decade period the effects of nerve agents were studied in hundreds of volunteer subjects. This chapter provides a history and overview of these studies and, although incomplete, furnishes a general description of the nature of those investigations. It is a tribute to those who conducted the investigations and to the stringent and well-controlled conditions under which they were conducted that so many subjects were exposed to these toxic materials with so few serious effects.

ACKNOWLEDGEMENTS

I thank Van M. Sim, MD, a leader and major investigator in the US effort in this program, for reviewing this chapter and for his helpful advice and comments.

I also thank Mr Patsy D'Eramo for library assistance in patiently locating and retrieving the old and obscure reports referenced.

REFERENCES

1. Koelle GB (1981) Organophosphate poisoning—an overview. *Fund Appl Toxicol*, **1**, 129–134.
2. The toxicity, symptoms, pathology, and treatment of T2104 poisoning in animals. Unpublished MOD report.
3. Sidell FR (1992) Clinical considerations in nerve agent intoxication. In: *Chemical Warfare Agents* (SM Somani, ed.), pp. 156–194. San Diego: Academic Press, Inc.
4. Eye effect of T.2104. Unpublished MOD report.
5. Tests of visual acuity affecting efficiency following exposure to a harassing dosage of tabun. Unpublished MOD report.
6. Report on exposures of unprotected men and rabbits to low concentrations of nerve gas vapour. Unpublished MOD report.

7. Harvey JC (1952) Clinical observations on volunteers exposed to concentrations of GB. *MLRR 114*.

8. Freeman G, Moore JC, Clanton BR *et al.* (1952) Observations on the effects of low concentrations of GB on man in rest and exercise. *MLRR 148*.

9. Cholinesterase as an aid to the early diagnosis of nerve gas poisoning. Part II: The variation of blood cholinesterases in man before and after the administration of very small quantities of G vapour by inhalation. Unpublished MOD report.

10. Grob D and Harvey AM (1953) The effects and treatment of nerve gas poisoning. *Am J Med*, **14**, 52–63.

11. Grob D and Harvey JC (1958) Effects in man of the anticholinesterase compound sarin (isopropyl methyl phosphonofluoridate). *J Clin Invest*, **37**, 350–368.

12. Grob D (1956) The manifestations and treatment of poisoning due to nerve gas and other organic phosphate anticholinesterase compounds. *Arch Intern Med*, **98**, 221–239.

13. Freeman G, Marzulli FN, Craig AB *et al.* (1953) The toxicity of liquid GB applied to the skin of man. *MLRR 217*.

14. Marzulli FN and Williams MR (1953) Studies on the evaporation, retention and penetration of GB applied to intact human and intact and abraded rabbit skin. *MLRR 199*.

15. The percutaneous toxicity of the G-compounds. Unpublished MOD report.

16. Freeman G, Marzulli F, Craig AB and Trimble JR (1954) The toxicity of liquid GA applied to the skin of man. *MLRR 250*.

17. Neitlich H (1965) Effect of percutaneous GD on human subjects. *CRDL TM 2-21*.

18. Krackow EH and Fuhr I (1949) Toxicity of GA vapor by cutaneous absorption for monkey and man. *MDR 179*.

19. Psychological effects of a G-agent on men. Unpublished MOD report.

20. Psychological effects of a G-agent on men; second report. Unpublished MOD report.

21. Cognitive and emotional changes after exposure to GB. Unpublished MOD report.

22. Davy E and Grosser G (1959) Some effects of certain chemical agents on motor and mental performance. *CWL SP 2-20*.

23. Studies of psychomotor performance. The effect of GB. Unpublished MOD report.

24. Coombs AY and Freeman G (1954) Observations of the effects of GB on intellectual function in man. *MLRR 310*.

25. Physical performance following inhalation of GB. Unpublished MOD report.

26. The effects of a single exposure to GB (Sarin) on human physical performance. Unpublished MOD report.

27. The intercostal muscles and GB inhalation in man. Unpublished MOD report.

28. The action of anticholinesterases and pressor amines on the capacity veins of the leg. Unpublished MOD report.

29. Changes in cardiac output following the administration of sarin and other pharmacological agents. Part 3. Human experiments using the low frequency critically damped ballistocardiograph. Unpublished MOD report.

30. GB exposure during simultaneous experimental acclimatization to heat and cold in man. Unpublished MOD report.

31. Detection of the 'G' gases by smell. Unpublished MOD report.

32. Dutreau CW, McGrath FP and Bray EH (1950) Toxicity studies on GD. 1. Median lethal concentration by inhalation in pigeons, rabbits, rats and mice. 2. Median detectable concentration by odor for man. *MDRR 8*.

33. McGrath FP, vonBerg VJ and Oberst FW (1953) Toxicity and perception of GF vapor. *MLRR 185*.

34. Cresthull P and Oberst FW (1964) Hazard to masked men eating and drinking in a sarin-contaminated atmosphere. *Armed Forces Chem J*, 21–23.

35. Cooper DY and Maloney JV Jr (1951) The pulmonary effects of inhalation of low concentrations of GB in man. *MLRR 82*.

36. Clements JA, Moore JC, Johnson RP and Lynott J (1952) Observations on airway resistance in men given low doses of GB by chamber exposure. *MLRR 122.*

37. An evaluation of the functional changes produced by the inhalation of GB vapour. Unpublished MOD report.

38. Air-way resistance changes in men exposed to GB vapour. Unpublished MOD report.

39. The single breath administration of sarin. Unpublished MOD report.

40. The intrabronchial distribution of soluble vapours at selected rates of gas flow. Unpublished MOD report.

41. The retention of inhaled GB vapour. Unpublished MOD report.

42. Ainsworth M and Shephard RJ (1961) The intrabronchial distribution of soluble vapours at selected rates of gas flow. In: *Inhaled Particles and Vapors* (CN Davies, ed.), pp. 233–247. New York: Pergamon Press.

43. Oberst FW, Koon WS and Crook JW (1952) Methods for quantitative determination of GB absorbed from inspired air of man during rest and exercise. *MLRR 143.*

44. Oberst FW, Crook JW, Christensen MK *et al.* (1959) Inhaled GB retention studies in man at rest and during activity. *CWLR 2296.*

45. Oberst FW, Koon WS, Christensen MK *et al.* (1968) Retention of inhaled sarin vapor and its effect on red blood cell cholinesterase activity in man. *Clin Pharmacol Ther*, **9**, 421–427.

46. Oberst FW (1961) Factors affecting inhalation and retention of toxic vapors. In: *Inhaled Particles and Vapours* (CN Davies, ed.), pp. 249–265. New York: Pergamon Press.

47. Brown ES (1957) Distribution of GB absorbed by oral inhalation. *CWL TM 22-1.*

48. The effects of a minor exposure to GB on military efficiency. Unpublished MOD report.

49. The effects of atropine and wearing respirators on the military efficiency of troops exposed to GB. Unpublished MOD report.

50. Johns RJ (1952) The effects of low concentrations of GB on the human eye. *MLRR 100.*

51. Effect on pupil size of exposure to GB vapor. Unpublished MOD report.

52. Estimation of the concentrations of nerve agent vapour required to produce measured degrees of miosis in rabbit and human eyes. Unpublished MOD report.

53. The effects of a chemical agent on the eyes of aircrew. Unpublished MOD report.

54. Moylan-Jones R and Price-Thomas DA (1973) Cyclopentolate in treatment of sarin miosis. *Br J Pharmacol*, **48**, 309–313.

55. Rubin LS and Goldberg MN (1957) The effect of GB on dark adaptation in man. III. The effect of tertiary and quaternary atropine salts on absolute scotopic threshold changes engendered by GB. *CWL TR 2155.*

56. Rubin LS and Goldberg MN (1958) Effect of tertiary and quaternary atropine salts on absolute scotopic threshold changes produced by an anticholinesterase (Sarin). *J Appl Physiol*, **12**, 305–310.

57. Rubin LS and Goldberg MN (1957) Effect of sarin on dark adaptation in man: threshold changes. *J Appl Physiol*, **11**, 439–444.

58. Rubin LS, Krop S and Goldberg MN (1957) Effect of sarin on dark adaptation in man: mechanism of action. *J Appl Physiol*, **11**, 445–449.

59. A comparative study of central visual field changes induced by GB (isopropylmethyl-phosphonofluoridate) vapours and physostigmine salicylate eyedrops. Unpublished MOD report.

60. Gazzard MF and Price-Thomas D (1975) A comparative study of central visual field changes induced by sarin vapour and physostigmine eye drops. *Exp Eye Res*, **20**, 15–21.

61. Stewart WC, Madill HAD and Dyer AM (1968) Night vision in the miotic eye. *Can Med Assoc J*, **99**, 1145–1148.

62. Sidell FR (1974) Soman and sarin: clinical manifestations and treatment of accidental poisoning by organophosphates. *Clin Toxicol*, **7**, 1–17.

63. Rengstorff RH (1985) Accidental exposure to sarin: vision effects. *Arch Toxicol*, **56**, 201–203.

64. Sidell FR and Groff WA (1974) The reactivatibility of cholinesterase inhibited by VX and sarin in man. *Toxicol Appl Pharmacol*, **27**, 241–252.

65. Ketchum JS, Sidell FR, Crowell EB Jr *et al.* (1973) Atropine, scopolamine, and ditran: comparative pharmacology and antagonists in man. *Psychopharmacology*, **28**, 121–145.

66. Kimura KK, McNamara BP and Sim VM (1960) Intravenous administration of VX in man. *CRDLR 3017*.

67. Sidell FR (1967) Human responses to intravenous VX. *EATR 4082*.

68. Sidell FR, Aghajanian GK and Groff WA (1973) The reversal of anticholinergic intoxication in man with the cholinesterase inhibitor VX. *Proc Soc Exp Biol Med*, **144**, 725–730.

69. Cresthull P, Koon WS, Musselman NP *et al.* (1963) Percutaneous exposure of the arm or the forearm of man to VX vapor. *CRDLR 3176*.

70. Human exposure to VX vapour. Unpublished MOD report.

71. Recovery of blood cholinesterase in man after exposure to VX. Unpublished MOD report.

72. Sim VM and Stubbs JL (1960) VX percutaneous studies in man. *CRDLR 3015*.

73. Sim VM (1962) Variability of different intact human-skin sites to the penetration of VX. *CRDLR 3122*.

74. Passage of VX through human skin. Unpublished MOD report.

75. Lubash GD and Clark BJ (1960) Some metabolic studies in humans following percutaneous exposure to VX. *CRDLR 3033*.

76. Vocci FJ, Hickman WE, Mehlman MA *et al.* (1959) The effect of n-octylamine on the penetration of VX by the percutaneous route in man. *CWL TM*, 24–22.

77. Cummings EG and Craig FN (1965) Effect of environment temperature on the penetration of VX applied to the cheek. *CRDLR 3256*.

78. Craig FN, Cummings EG, Mounter LA *et al.* (1967) Penetration of VX applied to the forearm at environmental temperatures of 65° and 115°F. *EATR 4064*.

79. Craig FN, Cummings EG and Sim VM (1977) Environmental temperature and the percutaneous absorption of a cholinesterase inhibitor, VX. *J Invest Dermatol*, **68**, 357–361.

80. Penetration of VX through clothing. Unpublished MOD report.

81. Sim VM, McClure C Jr, Vocci FJ *et al.* (1964) Tolerance of man to VX-contaminated water. *CRDLR 3231*.

82. Sidell FR and Groff WA (1966) Oral toxicity of VX to humans. *EATR 4009*.

83. Bowers MB Jr, Goodman E and Sim VM (1964) Some behavioral changes in man following anticholinesterase administration. *J Nerv Ment Dis*, **138**, 383–389.

84. Koon WS, Cresthull P, Crook JW *et al.* (1959) Odor detection of VX vapor with and without a stabilizer. *CWLR 2292*.

85. Sidell FR, Groff WA and Vocci F (1965) Effects of EA 3148 administered intravenously to humans. *CRDL TM 2-31*.

86. Craig AB and Woodson GS (1959) Observations on the effects of exposure to nerve gas. I. Clinical observations and cholinesterase depression. *Am J Med Sci*, **238**, 13–17.

87. Gaon MD and Werne J Report of a study of mild exposures to GB at Rocky Mountain Arsenal. *Medical Department US Army*. Undated report.

88. Holmes JH, Vincent T, Gingrich F and Gaon M (1958) Final progress report. *Contract Progress Report* DA-18-108-M-5586.

89. Lekov D, Dimitrov V and Mizkow Z (1966) Clinical observations of individuals contaminated by a pinacolic ester of methylfluorophosphine acid (soman). *Voenno Meditsinsko Delo*, **4**, 47–52.

90. Jager BV (1957) Case of GB poisoning. *Contract Progress Report* DA 18-108-CML-5421.

91. Brown EC Jr (1948) Effects of G agents on man: clinical observations. *MDR 158*.
92. Gammill JF, Gibson JDS and Cutuly E (1954) Report of mild exposure to GB in 21 persons. *DPG-MIB SR-1*.
93. Seed JC (1952) An accident involving vapor exposure to a nerve gas. *MLRR 146*.
94. Craig AB and Freeman G (1953) Clinical observations on workers accidentally exposed to 'G' agents. *MLRR 154*.
95. Craig AB Jr and Cornblath M (1953) Further clinical observations on workers accidentally exposed to G agents. *MLRR 234*.
96. Grob D and Johns RJ (1956) Effects of V-agent organic phosphate anticholinesterase compound EA 1508 in man following accidental exposure. *CWLR 2004*.
97. Brody BB (1954) Seventy five cases of accidental nerve gas poisoning at Dugway Proving Ground. *DPG-MIB SR-5*.
98. Freeman G, Hilton KC and Brown ES (1956) V poisoning in man. *CWLR 2025*.
99. Bertino JR, Geiger LE and Sim VM (1957) Accidental V-agent exposures. *CWLR 2156*.
100. Ward JR, Gosselin R, Comstock J *et al.* (1952) Case report of a severe human poisoning by GB. *MLRR 151*.
101. Ward JR (1962) Case report: exposure to a nerve gas. In: *Artificial Respiration. Theory and Applications* (JL Whittenberger, ed.), pp. 258–265. New York: Harper and Row.

6

MUSTARD GAS

'Mustard gas' is a misnomer. The compound usually referred to as mustard gas is sulphur mustard: a liquid which boils at 217°C. Both liquid sulphur mustard and the vapour given off are vesicant, i.e. produce blistering. Many mustard compounds other than sulphur mustard have been examined for their potential as chemical warfare agents. During World War II several hundred mustard-related compounds were synthesized. Of these, the nitrogen mustards and sesqui mustard have attracted some attention. Only sulphur mustard has been used on a large scale in war. Several of the nitrogen mustards have found peaceful uses as antimitotic agents used in the treatment of various cancers. In the following account mustard gas should be taken as indicating sulphur mustard.

HISTORICAL ASPECTS

The exact date of the first synthesis of sulphur mustard seems to be unknown: 1820, 1822 and 1854 have all been quoted by various writers. West[1] reported that Despretz recorded the formation of a disagreeably smelling compound produced by the action of ethylene on sulphur chloride. Niemann and Guthrie separately synthesized and described the properties of sulphur mustard in 1860. Niemann's description is accurate and is given below:

> The characteristic property of this oil is also a very dangerous one. It consists of the fact that the minutest trace which may accidentally come into contact with any portion of the skin, though at first causing no pain, produces in the course of a few hours a reddening and on the following day a severe blister which suppurates for a long time and is very difficult to heal.[1]

This description, written 135 years ago, would be difficult to improve upon today. Synthesis of pure sulphur mustard was reported by Victor Meyer.[2]

The development of sulphur mustard as a chemical warfare agent was undertaken by Fritz Haber in Germany during World War I, and mustard was used for the first time on the night of 12 July 1917 at Ypres.[3] British forces were the first to be exposed to mustard gas, and during the first three months of use more than 14 000 British casualties were produced. By the end of the war more than 120 000 British mustard gas casualties had occurred. Some writers have put the total number of mustard gas casualties produced during World War I as high as 400 000. The mortality rate amongst mustard casualties was low: 2–3%.[4]

It is not widely known that British interest in mustard gas preceded its use by German forces. Sir Charles Lovatt Evans[5] worked on chemical warfare agents during World War I and it has been recorded in a biographical memoir that:

> in January 1916 Lovatt Evans joined the RAMC and was seconded to work at The Royal Army Medical College of Millbank where Starling, with the rank of Major was in charge of the Anti-Gas Department. There they studied arsine, phosgene, hydrocyanic acid and mustard gas, the last at the suggestion of Harold W Dudley, and Starling advised its use but it was rejected. Lovatt Evans recalled that 'when, some fifteen months later mustard gas was used by the Germans, Starling was infuriated and made a vigorous protest at the highest level; the result of this was that he was promoted to Lt Col and sent to Salonika as Army Chemical Adviser, with nothing particular to do. He did it very well and was awarded a CMG....'

The effectiveness of mustard gas was greater than that of all the other chemical warfare agents used during World War I, and it came to be known as the 'King of Gases' or the 'King of the Battle Gases'.

Italian forces used sulphur mustard against Ethiopian forces in 1936 and it was used by Japanese forces against Chinese troops during World War II.[6] In the Iran–Iraq war, allegations, which proved well founded, of the use of sulphur mustard by Iraq were made.[7–9] In 1986, more than 30 Iranian casualties whose injuries were compatible with exposure to mustard gas were evacuated to London for treatment. The author was thus able to gather first-hand experience of treating mustard gas casualties.

Sulphur mustard has been little used in clinical medicine, the first report of its use being that of Adair.[10] Until recently, sulphur mustard was available for use in the treatment of psoriasis: Psoriasin marketed by Malco.[11] For an account of the effects of Psoriasin on the liver see Ciszewka-Popiolek et al.[12]

The name mustard was given to the compound by soldiers during World War I because of its smell. Some have described the smell as being similar to that of garlic, mustard, horse radish or leeks. Sulphur mustard should not be confused with mustard oil, allyl isothiocyanate, which, interestingly, is also a vesicant.[11] Sulphur mustard is often referred to in military manuals as H; this may be an abbreviated or generalized form of HS, said to stand for Hunstoffe. HN is sometimes used to denote nitrogen mustard (see below). During World War I, German forces referred to sulphur mustard as LOST, derived from the first letters of the names of the German chemists involved in its synthesis: Lommel and Steinkopf. The first use of sulphur mustard at Ypres led to French forces referring to it as Yperite. German shells containing sulphur mustard were marked with a yellow cross.

It may be thought that the details of the toxicity of a chemical warfare agent such as sulphur mustard represent a rather esoteric branch of toxicology: they do. However, civilian cases of exposure to sulphur mustard do occur. In 1984, some 23

Baltic fishermen showed effects of exposure to sulphur mustard as a result of mustard-gas-containing shells being caught in nets.[13] More than 50 000 tons of German chemical warfare munitions were dropped into the Baltic at the end of World War II by Allied forces. It is likely that these shells will continue to be recovered and will remain dangerous for many years yet.

PHYSICAL AND CHEMICAL PROPERTIES OF SULPHUR MUSTARD

The chemical structure of sulphur mustard is shown in Figure 1, and the physical characteristics are shown in Table 1.

The vapour pressure and volatility of mustard have been discussed in Chapter 2. For reference, Prentiss's table of vapour pressure and volatility is reproduced here in Table 2.

Sulphur mustard is hydrolysed by water according to the reaction:

$$(CH_2CH_2Cl)_2S + 2H_2O \rightarrow (CH_2CH_2OH)_2S + 2HCl$$

It should be noted that the vapour of sulphur mustard is 5.5 times as heavy as air and thus the gas will accumulate in shell craters and trenches.

The half-life for the hydrolysis of sulphur mustard by water has been reported as about 3–5 min. Such a figure is in practice misleading: sulphur mustard is rather immiscible with water and mixing is necessary for hydrolysis to take place. Sulphur mustard placed upon the ground will persist for a long period if protected from wind and rain. Persistence of quantities of sulphur mustard likely to be encountered in chemical warfare for 2–3 days is not unlikely. Increased temperature and pH increase the rate of hydrolysis. Oxidizing agents react with sulphur mustard to produce the corresponding sulphoxide and the sulphone (Figure 2). The sulphone is produced by stronger oxidizing agents, e.g. hypochlorite, and is itself a vesicant and may produce lacrimation and sneezing (it is described, therefore, as a sternutator, from the Latin *sternuo*: I sneeze). The sulphoxide is not a vesicant. These effects are not commonly observed by people working with the sulphone, because of its low vapour pressure. Sulphur mustard also reacts with free chlorine provided by compounds such as dichloramine, as shown in Figure 3.

Sulphur mustard is soluble in water to the extent of less than 0.1%, but is freely soluble in many common organic solvents, including ethanol, ether and chloroform. The vapour given off by a quantity of liquid sulphur mustard has considerable penetrating powers, rapidly passing through clothing and damaging the skin beneath.

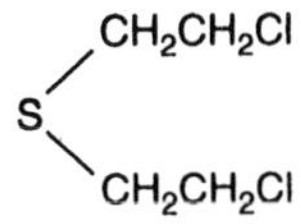

$$S\begin{cases} CH_2CH_2Cl \\ CH_2CH_2Cl \end{cases}$$

Figure 1. Sulphur mustard

Table 1. Physicochemical characteristics of sulphur mustard

Appearance	Yellow-brown oily liquid
Melting point	14.4°C
Boiling point	228°C (sometimes given as 217°C)
Specific gravity	1.27
Vapour density	5.4
Vapour pressure	
10°C	0.032 mmHg
25°C	0.112 mmHg
40°C	0.346 mmHg
Smell	Garlic, mustard, leeks

Table 2.

Temperature		Vapour pressure (mmHg)	Volatility (mg l^{-1})
°C	°F		
0	32	0.0260	0.250
5	41	0.0300	0.278
10	50	0.0350	0.315
15	59	0.0417	0.401
20	68	0.0650	0.625
25	77	0.0996	0.958
30	86	0.1500	1.443
35	95	0.2220	2.135
40	104	0.4500	3.660

Dichloroethylsulphoxide   Dichloroethylsulphone

Figure 2. Sulphoxide and sulphone of sulphur mustard

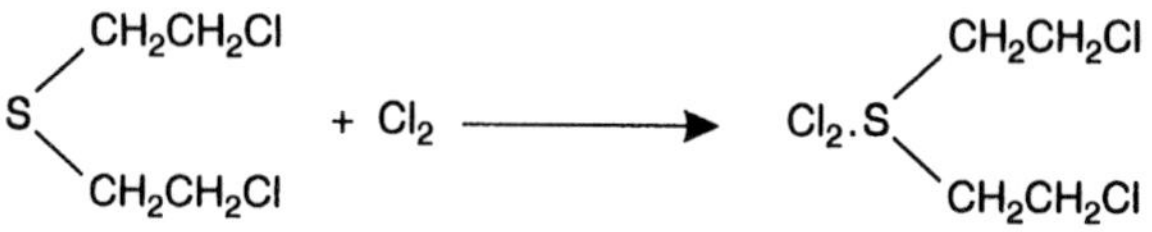

Tetrachloroethylsulphide

Figure 3. Reaction of sulphur mustard with free chlorine

Substances such as metal, glass and glazed tiles are generally impervious to mustard, though painted surfaces may take up vapour. This may be released later from the surface as the local ambient concentration of sulphur mustard vapour falls. Decontamination of painted surfaces is therefore important.

Sulphur mustard decomposes at high temperatures to produce toxic compounds, including active lacrimators: disposal of material contaminated with mustard by burning should, therefore, be undertaken with care.

PHYSICAL AND CHEMICAL PROPERTIES OF THE NITROGEN MUSTARDS

There are several nitrogen mustards. Those of relevance here are:

- HN_1: N-ethyl-2,2'-di(chloroethyl)amine
- HN_2: N-methyl-2,2'-di(chloroethyl)amine
- HN_3: 2,2',2''-tri(chloroethyl)amine

The chemical structures of the nitrogen mustards are shown in Figure 4, and the physicochemical characteristics are shown in Table 3.

Of the nitrogen mustards, HN_2 is familiar as the antimitotic agent mustine hydrochloride or mechlorethamine. From a military standpoint, HN_3 is the major representative of the nitrogen mustards.

LIKELY MODE OF EXPOSURE TO MUSTARD GAS

Sulphur mustard may be used as a chemical warfare agent in a number of ways. It may be delivered by artillery shell, rocket, bomb or aircraft spray. The agent is persistent and under cold conditions long-term contamination of ground may occur. Adequately protected troops would be expected to withstand well an attack with mustard gas. Precautions should be taken to ensure that protected troops do not carry mustard, for example on boots, into designated 'clean areas'.

Contamination of snow by mustard gas presents serious problems. Sulphur mustard freezes at 14°C and detection systems relying on detection of vapour may fail. Carriage of contaminated snow into buildings and the later release of mustard

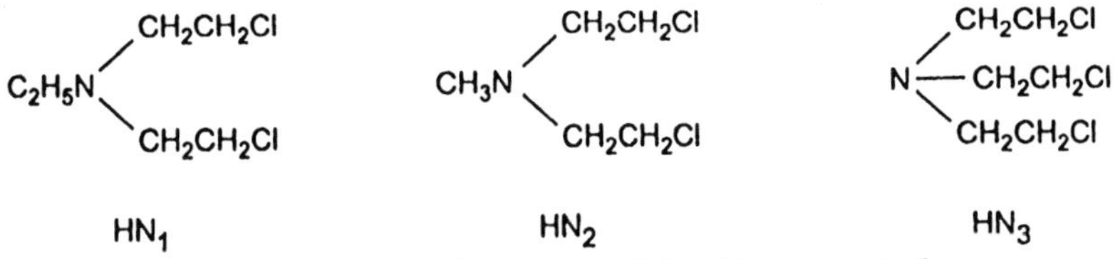

Figure 4. Chemical structures of the nitrogen mustards

Table 3. Physicochemical characteristics of the nitrogen mustards

Characteristic	HN_1	HN_2	HN_3
Appearance		Colourless or yellow oily liquid	
Melting point (°C)	− 34	− 60	− 4
Boiling point (°C)	85	75	138
Specific gravity	1.09	1.15	1.24
Vapour density	5.9	5.4	6.9
Vapour pressure			
10°C	0.0773	0.130	0.00272
25°C	0.2500	0.427	0.01090
40°C	0.7220	1.250	0.03820
Smell		Almost odourless; may smell of fish or soap	

vapour is a very real hazard for troops operating in an arctic climate. It is of interest that the freezing of mustard at the comparatively high temperature of 14°C led to difficulties in the design of artillery shells. Solidification of the contents of a shell were found to alter its ballistic properties, and solvents were added to prevent freezing. The use of chloropicrin for this purpose was developed by American experts. The mixture of phenyldichlorarsine with sulphur mustard to produce Winterlost has been mentioned in Chapter 2.

Mustard gas vapour will be carried long distances by wind. Prentiss[3] reported field tests which showed that:

> winds not exceeding 12 miles per hour, blowing over a normally saturated terrain, may transfer concentrations of mustard vapour sufficiently strong (0.070 mg per litre) to cause death within 30 minutes, for 500 to 1,000 yards downwind.

Naive troops or those equipped with inadequate protective equipment would not be expected to fare well if attacked with mustard.

Local contamination with sulphur mustard may extend to exposed water. Liquid mustard tends to sink as a heavy oily layer to the bottom of pools of water, leaving a dangerous oily film on the surface. Drinking from contaminated water sources may lead to damage to the gastrointestinal tract.

ABSORPTION OF SULPHUR MUSTARD, METABOLISM AND EXCRETION

Numerous studies of the penetration of skin by sulphur mustard have been undertaken. Accounts by Cullumbine[14] and Nagy[15] should be consulted for summaries of early studies. Renshaw demonstrated that 80% of a sample of liquid sulphur mustard placed upon the skin evaporated.[16] Of that penetrating the surface, about 10% was fixed to the skin, the remainder being absorbed systemically. This finding has been confirmed by recent studies[17,18] of the penetration by sulphur mustard through human foreskin grafted onto athymic nude mice (see below).

The rate of absorption of sulphur mustard across the human respiratory tract is unknown. Cameron *et al.*[19] demonstrated that some 80% of inhaled mustard was removed by the rabbit nasal mucosa. The corresponding figure for nitrogen mustard was 90%. Absorbed sulphur mustard binds rapidly to protein and disappears from the circulation.

A number of studies of the metabolism and excretion of sulphur mustard were prompted by the use of sulphur mustard in the Iran–Iraq war. Amongst these, those of Black *et al.* have been prominent.[20] It was shown that approximately 60% of an intraperitoneal dose of radiolabelled sulphur mustard was excreted by a rat within 24 h of administration. Some of the products excreted arose by hydrolysis of sulphur mustard but the majority were formed by conjugation with glutathione. The original paper should be consulted for details of the HPLC techniques used.

The relevance of studies of the metabolism of sulphur mustard conducted in rodents to clinical work may be questioned. In 1961, Davison reported studies of the metabolism of radiolabelled sulphur mustard in two patients suffering from terminal cancer.[21] Disappearance of sulphur mustard from the blood was rapid but excretion in urine was delayed as compared with that seen in rodents. This may have been due to kidney damage in these very ill patients. The importance of combination with glutathione was demonstrated in these studies.

TOXICITY OF SULPHUR MUSTARD

It was pointed out in Chapter 2 that the toxicity of chemical warfare agents should not be judged simply in terms of the doses or exposures necessary to cause death. Sulphur mustard is an effective incapacitating agent; indeed, its effectiveness in World War I rested on this property.

In the rat, the percutaneous LD_{50} is 9 mg kg^{-1}; corresponding figures for the dog and the rabbit are 20 and 100 mg kg^{-1}, respectively.

The percutaneous LD_{50} is not known in humans with any accuracy, though death is said to have occurred on exposure to 64 mg kg^{-1}.

Prentiss[3] gave the following figures for the toxicity of sulphur mustard:

- 0.15 mg l^{-1} is fatal on 10 min exposure
- 0.07 mg l^{-1} is fatal on 30 min exposure

Both Vedder[22] and Prentiss[3] placed great emphasis on the toxicity of sulphur mustard: Vedder pointed out that:

> In general, 0.07 mgm per litre may be considered as lethal for thirty minutes exposures, and it is therefore approximately five times more toxic than phosgene, which as we have seen is ten times as toxic as chlorine.

Effects upon the eyes

In humans the toxicity of mustard as regards effects of the vapour upon the eyes increases as the exposure is increased. In terms of Ct (mg min m^{-3}) the following may be used for guidance:

50 mg min m^{-3} Maximum safe exposure

70 mg min m^{-3} Mild reddening of the eyes

100 mg min m^{-3} Partial incapacitation due to eye effects

200 mg min m^{-3} Total incapacitation due to eye effects

It is important to note that 100 mg min m^{-3} is equivalent to an exposure to 0.0017 mg l^{-1} for 1 h. The odour of sulphur mustard is detectable at about 0.0013 mg l^{-1}.[3] The risk of incapacitation by conjunctivitis on exposure to levels of sulphur mustard vapour which would be difficult to detect by smell will be appreciated. Indeed, the risk is greater than these figures suggest: after initial exposure to sulphur mustard the sense of smell seems to be dulled and larger concentrations may be undetected. During World War I lacrimatory agents were often deployed with sulphur mustard to mask its smell.

Effects upon the skin

The effects of sulphur mustard upon the skin should be considered in terms of exposure to the agent in both liquid and vapour form.

LIQUID EXPOSURE

Exposure to 50 μg cm^{-2} for 5 min causes slight erythema, and exposure to 250–500 μg cm^{-2} for 5 min leads to blistering. As stated above, much of the applied sulphur mustard evaporates; regarding that which is absorbed, it has been said that as little as 6 μg cm^{-2} can cause blistering.[23]

VAPOUR EXPOSURE

The following may be used for guidance:

100–400 mg min m^{-3} Erythema of skin produced

200–1000 mg min m^{-3} Leads to blistering

750–1000 mg min m^{-3} Severe, incapacitating skin burns

The large range of values quoted for the effects of mustard vapour upon the skin takes into account the effects of ambient temperature. It was demonstrated during World War I that at higher ambient temperatures the effects of exposure to mustard vapour were very much more severe than those occurring at lower temperatures. At

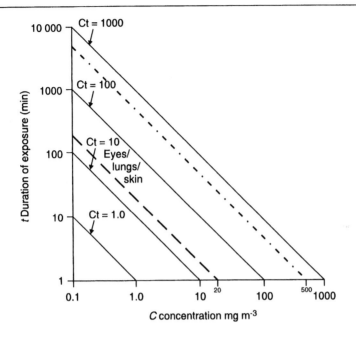

Figure 5. Effects of H: log–log plot of C and t. (---) $Ct = 20$ mg min m^{-3}; tolerable level? (-·-) $Ct = 500$ mg min m^{-3}; serious skin burns

an ambient temperature of 50°F, exposure to 1000 mg min m^{-3} of vapour may produce the same effects as exposure to 200 mg min m^{-3} of vapour at temperatures in excess of 80°F.

The effects of exposure to sulphur mustard vapour are shown in terms of concentration and time in Figure 5.

It will be realized that the figure is intended for guidance only: the likely inaccuracy of the predictions at the extremes of time and concentration will be obvious (Chapter 2).

TOXICITY OF HN$_2$ (MUSTINE HYDROCHLORIDE)

Because of its use in clinical practice, more is known about the toxicity of HN$_2$ than of the other nitrogen mustards. The effects of the accidental administration of 58 mg (instead of 5.8 mg) of HN$_2$ have been reported.[24] The patient was a 62-year-old woman suffering from Hodgkin's disease. Nine days after the dose the white cell count had fallen to 140 per mm^3. Haemoglobin fell to 8.2 g per 100 ml. Treatment with blood transfusions restored the red cell count and the patient was discharged on the 25th day after the accident. Some six months later she was readmitted with signs of a neurotoxic episode: confusion, ataxia, amnesia, headache, urinary incontinence, hyporeflexia and papilloedema. CAT scan revealed hydrocephalus of all cerebral ventricles. Recovery occurred over a period of 1 month. Late neurotoxic effects of nitrogen mustards are rare; early effects on the nervous system are more common.[25] Early clinical work with sulphur mustard does not yield comparable data: the drug tended to be applied directly to superficial tumours or by direct injection into tumours.

PHARMACOLOGY OF SULPHUR MUSTARD

Sulphur mustard is an alkylating agent: it forms covalent linkages with various nucleophilic cell constituents so that an alkyl group becomes attached.[26] The mode of action of the nitrogen mustards has been investigated in more detail than that of sulphur mustard, and excellent accounts are available.[27,28] Sulphur mustard and the nitrogen mustards are bifunctional alkylating agents in that the molecules possess two chains, each capable of undergoing the cyclization reactions necessary before alkylation can occur. Bifunctionality allows cross-linking of strands of nucleic acids by sulphur mustard, a key mechanism in producing cell damage. The reactions occurring in cross-linking of DNA are shown in Figure 6.

The binding of ethylenesulphonium ions, in the case of sulphur mustard, and ethylenimonium ions, in the case of nitrogen mustards, to DNA produces a range of effects, including the following:

- Alkylated guanine residues tend to form base pairs with thymine rather than cytosine, leading to coding errors and hence to inaccuracies in protein synthesis.
- Damaged guanine residues may be excised from the DNA molecule, leading to further damage.
- Two guanine residues may become cross-linked and produce major disruption in DNA functioning. This cross-linking is seen by some as the most serious of the effects of exposure to sulphur mustard.

Repair of DNA damage occurs in cells but this process can itself lead to further impairment of cell functioning. Polymerization of NAD under the influence of the poly(ADP-ribose) polymerase enzyme is an important part of the DNA repair process.[29] It has been suggested[17,18] that this process may lead to a damaging depletion of cellular levels of NAD.[30] Papirmeister proposed a biochemical hypothesis to explain the effects of sulphur mustard upon cells. In simplified form this ran as follows:

- Sulphur mustard alkylates purines in DNA, e.g. guanine.
- Apurinic endonucleases act at these sites, producing backbone breaks in DNA.
- The chromosomal enzyme poly(ADP-ribose) polymerase is activated.

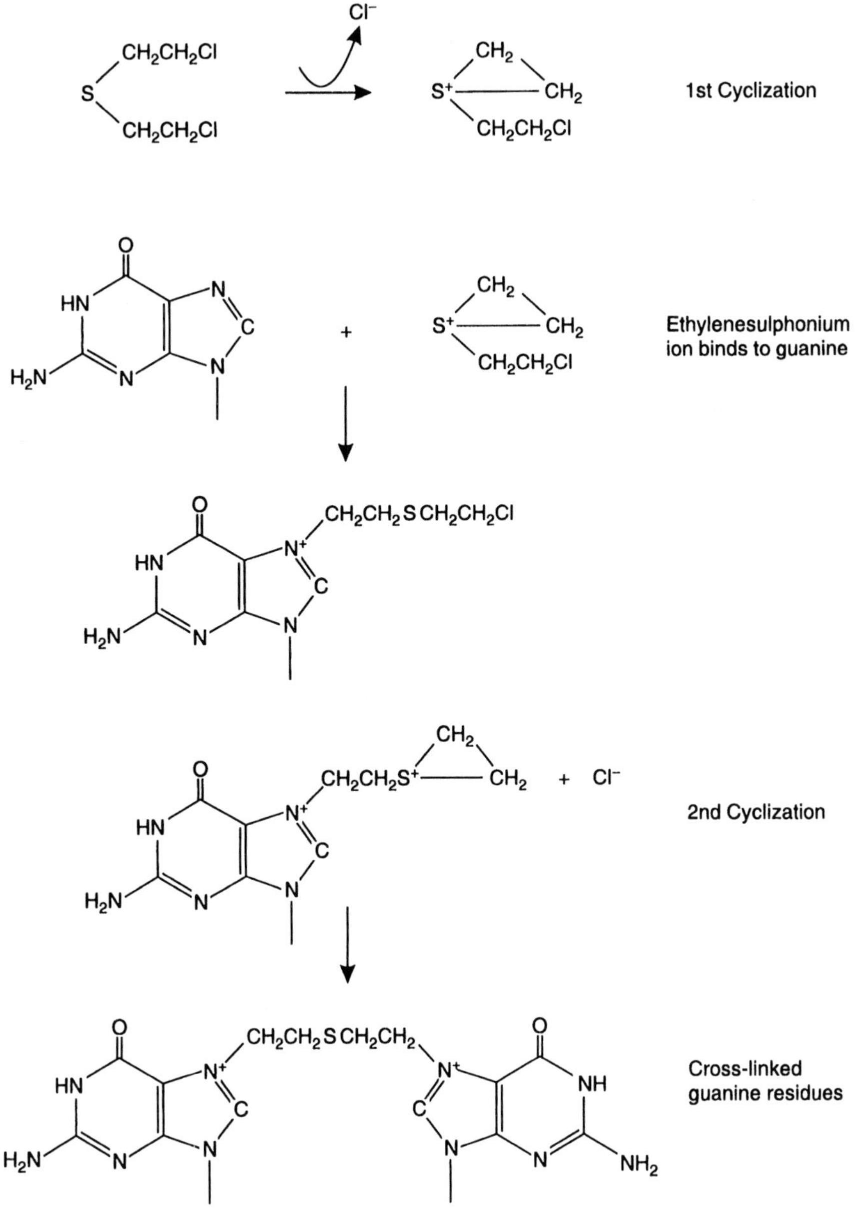

Figure 6. Reactions occurring in cross-linking of DNA

- NAD is utilized as a substrate and cellular levels of NAD fall.
- Glycolysis is inhibited.

This hypothesis was supported by early work which had demonstrated a good correlation between skin injury in experimental animals and inhibition of glycolysis.[31]

It should, however, be remembered that the exact link between chemical or biochemical damage by sulphur mustard and vesication remains elusive. The enhanced protease synthesis and release following DNA damage has been suggested as a means whereby the dermal–epidermal junction might be damaged and so lead to blistering.[32] This remains speculative. The remarkable lack of a clear understanding of the mechanism whereby sulphur mustard produces blistering should be seen in the context of other enigmas regarding the response of the skin to chemicals and physical insults. Concentrated acids and alkalis do not produce blistering, and near-fatal poisoning by barbiturates may produce blistering; of mammals, only human skin blisters on the application of sulphur mustard. This last observation is a cause of great surprise: however, the search for a suitable animal model for the effects of mustard gas upon skin has been long and intensive and, to date, unsuccessful. Application of sulphur mustard to the skin of young pigs and neonatal rats and mice[33] produces intradermal microblisters but the large pendulous fluid-filled blisters seen so commonly in mustard gas casualties seem to depend upon some property possessed only by human skin.

The effects of alkylating agents upon rapidly dividing tissues might be expected to be severe. Damage to the gut epithelium, hair loss and depression of bone marrow are all recognized side-effects of the clinical use of alkylating agents.

Both nitrogen and sulphur mustard have effects upon the central nervous system, including the induction of vomiting, nausea, convulsions and, in the case of nitrogen mustards, progressive muscular weakness. The cyclization of nitrogen mustard leads to the formation of a quaternary nitrogen grouping and this may account for the cholinomimetic effects sometimes reported after exposure: see Figure 7. The work of Hunt and Phillips[34] on the acute effects of nitrogen mustard (HN_2) should be consulted for details of the cholinomimetic effects.

HISTOPATHOLOGY OF SULPHUR MUSTARD EXPOSURE

The gross pathological effects of sulphur mustard exposure will be described in the section on clinical effects; here the account will be limited to the light and electron

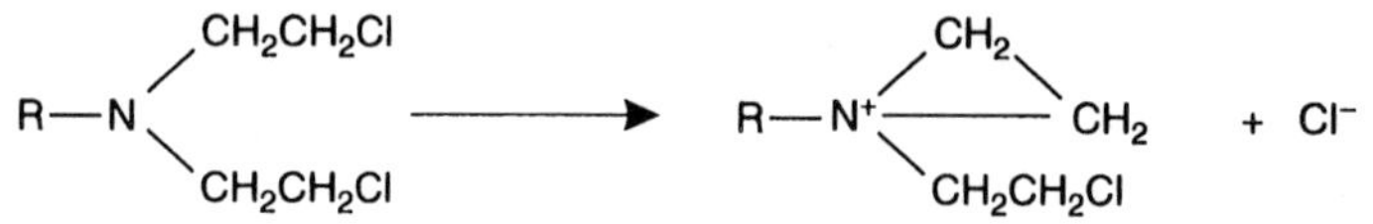

Figure 7.

microscopic appearances of damaged tissue. A very large number of experiments, using animal models and human volunteers, designed to investigate the effects of exposure to sulphur mustard were undertaken during World War I. These have been described in detail by Ireland.[35] Ireland's account is particularly valuable for the photographic material presented.

Skin effects

In one series of experiments sulphur mustard was applied in droplets of approximately 0.0004 cm^3, producing a 3–4-mm-diameter contamination to the skin of the forearm in a series of volunteers. The progress of the lesions was observed and histopathological studies were made by means of biopsy.

Thirty minutes after contamination the epidermis appeared generally shrunken with vacuolation of the deeper layers and nuclear changes in the granular layer. The cornified layer appeared rather thicker than usual and appeared to separate readily from the stratum lucidum. Occasional vacuoles were seen in the deepest layers of the epidermis. The dermis showed fewer changes than the epidermis.

Capillary damage in the papillary layer of the dermis was identified. The endothelial cells of capillaries in this region showed nuclear damage and vacuolation of their cytoplasm. Pericapillary oedema was noted. Leukocyte diapedesis was seen in some capillaries but near the centre of the lesion blood vessels appeared contracted and empty. Lymphatic vessels in the dermis were dilated.

The hair follicles and sebaceous glands showed changes similar to those described above, though sweat glands appeared normal.

By 18 h after contamination a typical vesicle had appeared. On microscopy, liquefaction and hydropic changes in the epithelium of the centre of the lesion were noted. Small vesicles were seen at the epidermal–dermal border and in some places the epidermis was separated from the dermis by fluid. Epithelial cells of hair follicles and sebaceous glands also showed these changes.

The upper part of the dermis appeared oedematous and contained many degenerating nuclei. Capillary damage and local oedema was also seen in this region. Deeper in the dermis blood vessels were congested and the lymphatic vessels appeared dilated and filled with proteinaceous fluid.

The subcutaneous tissues showed changes, particularly in relation to small blood vessels. Congestion of blood vessels and dilatation of lymphatics was commonly seen.

By thirty-six hours after contamination, almost complete epidermal destruction was observed. Such epidermal cells as were left showed pyknotic nuclei. In some areas only the deepest layer of epidermal nuclei remained. Leukocyte infiltration of the dermis was noted, particularly in relation to sweat glands, hair follicles and sebaceous glands. Small pockets of oedema and inflammatory cell infiltration were observed in the subcutaneous tissues.

The later progress of the lesion may be summarized as follows:

- 40–50 h: collapse of vesicles and progressive necrosis
- 72 h: eschar formation beginning
- 4–6 days: eschar beginning to slough
  oedema and hyperaemia persisting locally
- 19 days: separation of eschar, leaving a pigmented scar

The examination of human postmortem material during World War I produced further observations:

- Infection was often found, the associated inflammatory response being marked.
- Striking increases in pigmentation were recorded. Cells were seen to be laden with melanin and this occurred not only in the basal layer of the epidermis.
- Deep burning was associated with increased dermal fibroblast activity.
- Thrombosis of blood vessels was seen only in instances of very severe burns.

Small lesions were observed to heal slowly by centripetal spread of peripheral epidermal cells and dermal fibrosis if dermal damage had occurred. Again, the increase in melanin production was characteristic.

In 1984, Vogt reported a more detailed study using rabbits and guinea pigs.[36] The light microscopic features described above were confirmed and extended by electron microscopy and the following observations added.

Histochemical observations   There was an increase in acid phosphatase and arylsulphatase activity in the region of basal epidermal cells, reaching a maximum at 3 h post-exposure. This was attributed to activation of lysosomal enzymes. At 8 and 19 h post-exposure increased arylsulphatase staining of fibroblasts and histiocytes was noted. At 19 h clusters of large ATPase-positive mononuclear cells were identified just below the epidermis. These may have been derived from the Langerhans cells of the antigen-presenting series.

Vascular permeability studies   Evans blue and horse radish peroxidase were used as markers of vascular permeability. At high doses of sulphur mustard (250 μg cm^{-2}) an early (30–60 min post-exposure) capillary fluid leak was noted. This appeared to be a reversible phenomenon. Later, and at all doses, a more marked leak occurred (8–48 h post-exposure). The proposal that the early effect may have been due to direct effects of sulphur mustard on capillary endothelial cells and that the later leak might be local vasoactive metabolite dependent was put forward.

Healing pattern   The inflammatory response was seen to reach a peak at 24–72 h post-exposure. Healing took place over 10 days.

The two-stage effect proposed could be summarized:

1. Immediate phase (within first hour)—direct damage to endothelium of capillaries and to superficial fibroblasts.

2. Delayed phase—death of basal epidermal cells, generalized vascular leak, invasion by inflammatory cells.

It is interesting to note that the production of tissue oedema was inhibited by the application of topical steroids combined with systemic steroid therapy, but that by 48 h post-exposure no difference could be detected between the lesions of control- and steroid-treated animals. No evidence of enhanced healing of the lesions was obtained.

As has already been stated, animal skin does not blister as a result of contact with mustard. Papirmeister in 1984 reported an extensive investigation of the effects of sulphur mustard on human skin using an interesting animal/human model.[17] Athymic nude mice are immunologically incompetent and will accept skin grafts of human material. A similar rat model has also been developed. Human foreskin was used as the graft material. The most important findings reported from this study were probably those describing the pathological sequence at the electron microscopic level. The following sequence of changes was defined:

1. Condensation and margination of heterochromatin.
2. Loss of euchromatin.
3. Blebbing of nuclear membrane.
4. Appearance of perinuclear vacuoles.
5. Swelling of endoplasmic reticulum.
6. Progressive dissociation of rosettes of free ribosomes.
7. Formation of cytoplasmic vacuoles.
8. Loss of integrity of basal cell membrane.
9. Leakage of cell contents and debris into lamina lucida of the basement membrane.
10. Disruption of anchoring filaments of basal hemidesmosomes.
11. Phagocyte infiltration into areas of damage.

He also noted that not all basal epidermal cells were equally affected and suggested that the capacity for repair might be dependent on the stage of the cell cycle at the time of application of the mustard.

Sensitivity to sulphur mustard varies considerably from person to person. Also, some individuals seem to become sensitized to sulphur mustard. This was investigated by Sulzberger, who reported a wide range of dermatological reactions to sulphur mustard.[37] The authors' paper, which contains many interesting details relating to mustard gas and to other vesicants, should be consulted for details. Racial differences in sensitivity have been reported and disputed. Sulzberger reported that negroes were less sensitive to sulphur mustard than whites and considered the suggestion that blond people were more sensitive than dark-haired whites. The latter suggestion they could not confirm. The greater sensitivity of whites than negroes has also been questioned by later workers.

Eye effects of sulphur mustard

Detailed studies of the effects of sulphur mustard and other mustards upon the eyes have been reported by Mann, Warthin and Weller and Friedenwald *et al.*[38-40] The following account draws heavily upon Mann's seminal studies.

The effects of liquid sulphur mustard upon the eye mirror those upon the skin. Early corneal changes, including pyknosis in the epithelium and substantia propria, leading to corneal necrosis by 12 h, were reported. Regeneration of the cornea occurred by approximately 65 h post-exposure in animals. Vascularization and scarring of the cornea followed in more severe cases. Vapour exposure was less likely to produce permanent eye changes than liquid exposure. Corneal necrosis was uncommon in cases of vapour-only exposure.

Conjunctival changes, including necrosis, desquamation and marked oedema, were noted. Petechial haemorrhages were commonly seen. In very severe cases of exposure during World War I, iritis and iridocyclitis were seen. The extension of changes into the posterior chamber of the eye was rare. Accessory structures, including the lacrimal gland, showed increased function and some of the smaller glands inflammation and necrosis. Periorbital tissues often showed congestion and oedema, and a mild cellular infiltration of orbital muscles occurred. During World War I, secondary ophthalmic infections were comparatively common and panophthalmitis was seen.

One of the most distressing effects of exposure to sulphur mustard which appears after a considerable delay is late-onset blindness associated with keratitis of the cornea. This was reported in cases of World War I mustard exposure during the 1920s and 1930s; the exact explanation for this effect seems unclear. Damage to the nerve endings of the cornea reflected in corneal anaesthesia seems to play a part.

The conjunctival (and presumably corneal) effects of sulphur mustard are generally believed only to be produced when the eye has been exposed to either vapour or liquid. Warthin and Weller reported Haldane as claiming that subcutaneous injection of mustard could 'cause conjunctivitis and death from pneumonia owing to the reabsorption of the gas into the circulation'. These observations appeared to confirm those made by Victor Meyer but could not be confirmed by Warthin and Weller.[39]

Eye effects of nitrogen mustards

As far as the effects of 'mustards' upon the eye are concerned, two groups may be defined. These were identified by Mann[38] as:

1. The 'mustard gas group', comprising sulphur mustard and HN_3. HN_3 was observed to produce the same pattern of lesions as described for sulphur mustard above.
2. The 'nitrogen mustard group', comprising HN_1 and HN_2.

The term 'nitrogen mustard group' was coined by Ida Mann[38] during an extensive study of the eye effects of mustard compounds undertaken during World War II. It is confusing that HN_3 produced similar effects to sulphur mustard and therefore does not figure in the 'nitrogen mustard group'. The effects of the nitrogen mustard gas were described as follows:

> The typical reaction of the eye to injury with a compound of this class is characterised by the absence of a latent period and the depth of the injury due to a great power of penetration. The cornea is injured, the pupil contracts and a cellular exudate from the ciliary body appears within an hour.

Later changes included:

- haemorrhagic iridocyclitis
- corneal oedema and vascularization
- slow recovery
- recurrent intraocular haemorrhages
- depigmentation of the iris and cataract formation

Mann summed up:

> This reaction is typical and quite unlike that due to mustard gas, with its latent interval, absence of severe intraocular involvement and its typical relapsing vascularising keratitis.[38]

Respiratory changes

The extent of changes seen in the respiratory tract following exposure to sulphur mustard is dependent upon the duration of the exposure and the concentration of the agent in the inhaled air. Under warm environmental conditions the respiratory effects of sulphur mustard vapour were observed to be increased. Data collected during World War I are often difficult to interpret because of the high incidence of super-added infection in cases coming to postmortem examination.

UPPER RESPIRATORY TRACT

Necrosis of the epithelium of the larynx, trachea and bronchi commonly occurred in cases of severe exposure, a 'diphtheritic' membrane being seen in severe cases. Hyperaemia of and petechial haemorrhages in the surface layers were common in cases of less severe exposure. Similar erosions in experimental animals persisted for some months after exposure to the sulphur mustard. Occasionally during World War I gangrenous changes in the trachea were reported. At light microscopy an exudate of epithelial cells, fibrin and mucus was seen. The basement membrane appeared swollen and poorly defined. Oedema of subepithelial tissues associated with inflammatory cell infiltration and dilatation of blood vessels was common.

In more severe cases damage extended to the connective tissue and smooth muscle components of the walls of the airways.

During the reparative phase extensive squamous metaplasia was noted, the earliest changes being in the ducts of mucous glands. Cover of the entire damaged surface by a metaplastic stratified squamous epithelium was recorded. The later development of this epithelium is not well described and restoration of a pseudostratified ciliated columnar epithelium is not well documented.

CHANGES IN LUNG PARENCHYMA

Here the high incidence of secondary infection makes interpretation of postmortem findings particularly difficult. Even after low-dose exposures, congestion and oedema appeared to be present in some cases and secondary infection often occurred. Classical changes were associated with those areas of lung parenchyma close to the airways.

The peribronchial alveoli were seen to contain free red cells and often showed collapse. Further from the airways a fibrinous exudate rather than free blood filled the alveoli. The red peribronchial zone seen macroscopically usually extended some 2–3 mm from the bronchial wall. The hypothesis of diffusion of sulphur mustard through the bronchial wall was put forward to explain these effects.

Generalized areas of collapse, emphysema and oedema were all commonly seen at postmortem. During the reparative phase thickening of bronchial walls, organization of fibrinous oedema and proliferation of deeply staining cuboidal alveolar cells (type II cells) was recorded. These cells were seen to grow over plugs of fibrinous exudate. The final picture was one of an organizing chemical pneumonitis.

Study of tissue samples from lungs of Iranian casualties who died as a result of exposure to mustard gas has revealed a pattern identical with that described above. In all, tissue from four patients was studied. Alveolar capillary congestion, haemorrhage, oedema, the formation of hyaline membranes and fibrosis were seen. The casualties died as a result of multisystem organ failure and the changes in the lung parenchyma were very similar to those seen in cases of adult respiratory distress syndrome (ARDS).

Bone marrow changes

The effects of sulphur mustard upon the bone marrow were investigated during World War I by Pappenheimer and Vance.[41] Rabbits exposed to sulphur mustard at a level capable of inducing bone marrow depression revealed a general depletion of all elements of the bone marrow and a replacement by fat. The cells of the granulocyte series and the megakaryocytes appeared more susceptible to damage than those of the erythropoietic series.

During World War I careful studies were made of the changes in white blood cell (WBC) counts which occurred after exposure to mustard gas. The following phases were described:

1. Day 1 to day 3: an increase in WBC count in peripheral blood was noted. This was accounted for mainly by a great increase in circulatory polymorphs. Lymphocytes were reduced in numbers during this period.
2. From day 4 onwards: in severe cases a very rapid fall in the WBC count was recorded. Vedder[22] reported a WBC count of 33 800 on the second day, falling to 15 800 on the third day to 172 on the seventh day 6 h before death. The early leukocytosis and subsequent leukopaenia was observed in Iranian casualties seen during 1985 and 1986.

SYMPTOMS AND SIGNS OF SULPHUR MUSTARD POISONING

The use of mustard gas during the Iraq–Iran war furnished considerable clinical material and demonstrated that lessons forgotten since World War I regarding the management of chemical warfare casualties had to be relearnt. Colonel Jan L. Willems collected information on 65 casualties treated during the Iran–Iraq war in European hospitals. His report 'Clinical management of mustard gas casualties' should be studied by everyone who requires an up-to-date understanding of the effects of mustard gas.[42] It is particularly valuable for the photographs of lesions excellently reproduced in colour, which are more useful than black and white records of cases during World War I and are of perhaps even greater value than the coloured illustrations prepared by A.K. Maxwell during World War I. (A.K. Maxwell was a distinguished medical illustrator whose initials will be familiar to all who have studied the standard anatomical work, *Gray's Anatomy*.)

The hallmark of sulphur mustard exposure is the occurrence of a latent, symptom- and sign-free period of some hours post-exposure. The duration of this interval is dependent on the mode of exposure, on environmental temperature and probably on the individual. Some people are markedly more sensitive to mustard than others.

Table 4 shows the evolution of symptoms and signs which might be expected following a *severe* exposure to sulphur mustard vapour. Liquid exposure of the eyes will produce more severe, possibly permanent, eye damage.

If mustard-contaminated food or water are ingested, then the symptomatology will differ from that listed above and the onset, after a few hours, of nausea, vomiting, abdominal pain, bloody vomiting and diarrhoea (in cases of severe poisoning), shock and prostration may be expected.

Symptoms and signs associated with skin lesions

The sequence of skin changes normally seen is as follows:

1. Erythema (2–48 h post-exposure). This may be very striking and reminiscent of scarlet fever. Slight oedema of the skin may occur. Itching is common and may

Table 4. Development of symptoms and signs following severe exposure to mustard gas

Time post-exposure	Symptoms and signs
20–60 min	Nausea, retching, vomiting and eye smarting have all been *occasionally* reported. Often no signs or symptoms are produced
2–6 h	Nausea, fatigue, headache. Inflammation of eyes. Development of intense pain in eyes, lacrimation, blepharospasm, photophobia, rhinorrhoea
	Reddening of face and neck, soreness of throat. Voice becomes hoarse and may be lost completely. Increased pulse and respiratory rate
6–24 h	General increase in severity of above effects. Inflammation of inner thighs, genitalia, perineum, buttocks and axillae followed by blister formation. Blisters may be large, pendulous and filled with a clear, yellow fluid
Death within 24 h of exposure is very rare	
48 h	Condition generally worsened. Blistering more marked. Coughing appears: muco pus and necrotic slough may be expectorated. Intense itching of skin is common. Increase in skin pigmentation occurs

be intense. As the erythema fades, areas of increased pigmentation are left (this sequence is reminiscent of that seen in sunburn).

2. Blistering. The appearance of the blisters has been described above. Blisters are not painful *per se*, though they may be uncomfortable and may feel tense. Blisters at points of flexure, anterior aspects of elbows and posterior aspects of knees can seriously impede movement. Mustard blisters are delicate and may be easily rubbed off by contact with bed linen or bandages or during transport of casualties. Crops of new blisters may appear as late as the second week post-exposure. The author has seen a blister about 1.5 × 0.5 cm in size on the thigh of an Iranian mustard gas casualty as late as approximately 3 weeks post-exposure. By this time, of the patient's earlier symptoms and signs, only mild photophobia and some darkening of the skin remained.

   Blister fluid is not dangerous and does not produce secondary blistering if applied to skin.[37]

   This last observation has been a cause of considerable controversy. In 1943 Sulzberger and Katz performed a definitive experiment in which blister fluid from blisters produced upon volunteers by sulphur mustard and also lewisite was aspirated and applied to normal skin both of the blistered individual and others. No blistering was produced by the application of the blister fluid.[43]

3. Deep burning leading to full-thickness skin loss: this is particularly likely to occur on the penis and scrotum.

PROGRESS OF LESIONS

Though blisters are, as has already been pointed out, painless, once the blister cover is lost the lesions tend to be painful and some patients complain of very severe pain. Healing of skin lesions is slow. The areas which were markedly erythematous darken and may become very hyperpigmented. Brownish-purple to black discoloration of some areas may occur. This last change was particularly marked in some Iranian casualties and was commented upon by Willems.[42] These changes tend to disappear over a period of several weeks, with desquamation leading to the appearance of areas of hypopigmentation. The appearance of such areas alongside those of hyperpigmentation may be striking.

Experience in 1986 of Iranian mustard gas casualties suggested that hyperpigmentation was most marked at the margins of affected areas. In some the pigmentation seen was uneven and suggested, to some, droplet contamination. This was later doubted on the grounds that liquid contamination would be expected to produce more severe skin effects than were observed in these areas. The increases in pigmentation seen in several diseases and conditions are incompletely understood; for example, chronic arsenic poisoning produces hyperpigmentation and hypopigmentation which is classically described as having a 'raindrop' pattern. Why the pigmentation should occur in such a pattern seems to be unknown.

Rubbing the damaged skin of patients exposed to mustard can lead to the production of secondary blisters (Nikolsky's sign: this sign can also be elicited in cases of pemphigus vulgaris). The late blistering described above is probably a manifestation of this rather than a delayed effect of sulphur mustard itself.

Willems has commented upon attempts to correlate the extent of the skin lesions with the severity of the intoxication.[42] This proved very difficult, and the presence or absence of pulmonary damage and leukopaenia proved a better guide to the degree of poisoning.

Symptoms and signs associated with eye lesions

A marked conjunctivitis, local oedema, including oedema of the eyelids, blepharospasm and lacrimation are the classical signs. To these may be added early miosis, photophobia and severe eye pain (the headache sometimes described may be related to the eye pain and miosis). The onset of conjunctivitis may be delayed for up to 48 h in cases of mild exposure. Later adherence of the follicular margins with a mucoserous discharge occurs. As this dries, crusting is produced.

If the damaged eye is opened for examination (this may be very painful) a hyperaemic band may be identified crossing the globe horizontally. This observation made during World War I was confined to cases seen in the early stages. Later, a white band reflecting severe damage replaces the hyperaemic band. Corneal ulceration is said to be unusual in cases of vapour exposure. However, postmortem examination of the eye of an Iranian casualty who had been exposed to mustard vapour in 1986 revealed stripping of the corneal epithelium. In cases of severe exposure, mustard may penetrate the anterior chamber and adhesion of the iris to the lens capsule may occur.

Infection of the eye is a very serious consequence of mustard gas exposure and may produce blindness.

Symptoms and signs associated with lesions of the respiratory tract

Rhinorrhoea, often profuse, is commonly seen after vapour exposure. Epistaxis may occur in severely affected patients. Inflammation and ulceration of the palate, nasopharynx, oropharynx and larynx follow, the voice becomes hoarse and temporary aphonia may occur. Reports from World War I suggest that laryngeal oedema and/or spasm sufficiently severe to necessitate tracheostomy occurred very seldom.

Willems[42] reported findings on bronchoscopy in two patients: bilateral erythematous inflammation of the mucosa with bleeding and purulent secretions were reported. Casts of necrotic sloughed mucosa were also seen.

Coughing may be severe. As stated, a mucopurulent expectorate is produced. Necrotic slough may also be produced.

During World War I, factory workers involved in the production of mustard gas were particularly at risk. It was reported[44] that:

> At the main British factory, there were 1400 casualties among the plant workers, the accidentally burned and blistered exceeding 100 per cent of the staff every three months (presumably some members of staff were injured more than once). Conditions at the principal French plant, which supplied three quarters of the Allied-fired mustard gas, were equally unpleasant: The personnel ... is 90 per cent voiceless. About 50 per cent cough continuously.... By long exposure to the small amounts of vapour constantly in the air of the work rooms, the initial resistance of the skin is finally broken down. The chief result is that the itch makes sleep nearly impossible and the labourers are very much run down.

Non-specific symptoms of mustard gas poisoning

Though the symptoms and signs listed above are the classical signs of sulphur mustard poisoning, clinicians should be aware of a group of symptoms and signs reported during World War I and not yet adequately explained. These included:

- diffuse skin pigmentation (this has been mentioned above)
- hypotension
- marked apathy and asthenia
- mental disturbance

The suggestion of adrenal damage was made during World War I to explain some of these effects. This has not been confirmed.

In 1986, Norris reviewed a number of aspects of the effects of mustard gas and reported work done in the late stages of World War I on the 'functional neurosis' which some authors claimed was recognized in 22% of all mustard cases.[45] He commented:

> They described an anxiety state in mild cases of gas poisoning and coughing or photophobia reinforced by hysteria and they produced the following breakdown of the 22% of casualties with neurosis:
>
> Functional photophobia 12.6% of all cases
>
> Functional aphonia 7.2%
>
> Functional vomiting 1.0%
>
> Effort syndrome 1.2%
>
> ('functional' in this context implies absence of a clear pathological mechanism, at least of a physical kind).

FIRST-HAND ACCOUNT OF EFFECTS OF MUSTARD GAS

1. Reported by Victor Lefebure 1921 from an account provided by a casualty.[46]

> I was gassed by dichlor-diethyl sulphide, commonly known as mustard stuff, on July 22 [1917]. I was digging in [Livens Projectors] to fire on Lombartzyde. Going up we met a terrible strafe of HE and gas shells at Nieuport. When things quietened a little I went up with the three GS wagons, all that were left, and the carrying parties. I must say that the gas was clearly visible and had exactly the same smell as horseradish. It had *no* immediate effect on the eyes or throat. I suspected a delayed action and my party all put their masks on.
>
> On arriving at the emplacement we met a very thick cloud of the same stuff drifting from the front line system. As it seemed to have no effect on the eyes I gave orders for all to put on their mouthpieces and noseclips so as to breathe none of the stuff, and we carried on.
>
> Coming back we met another terrific gas shell attack at Nieuport. Next morning, myself and all the eighty men we had up there were absolutely blind. The horrid stuff had a delayed action on the eyes, causing temporary blindness some seven hours afterwards. About 3,000 were affected. One or two of our party never recovered their sight and died. The casualty clearing stations were crowded. On August 3, with my eyes still very bloodshot and weak and wearing blue glasses, I came home and went into Millbank Hospital on August 15.

2. In October 1918 Adolf Hitler was exposed to mustard gas. He was at the time a runner in the 16th Bavarian Reserve Regiment. He included the following graphic account in *Mein Kampf* (Vol. 1, 1924).

> During the night of October 13–14th [1918] the British opened an attack with gas on the front south of Ypres. They used the yellow gas whose effect was unknown to us, at least from personal experience. I was destined to experience it that very night. On a hill

south of Werwick, in the evening of 13 October, we were subjected to several hours of heavy bombardment with gas bombs, which continued through the night with more or less intensity. About midnight a number of us were put out of action, some for ever. Towards morning I also began to feel pain. It increased with every quarter of an hour, and about seven o'clock my eyes were scorching as I staggered back and delivered the last dispatch I was destined to carry in this war. A few hours later my eyes were like glowing coals, and all was darkness around me.

This excellent description highlights the delayed effect of mustard gas upon the eyes and also the pain and incapacitation associated with such injuries. Hitler's reluctance to use chemical weapons during World War II has been attributed by some, perhaps fancifully, to his experience recorded above.

CLINICAL CHEMISTRY AND OTHER INVESTIGATIONS

Vesicles may be aspirated and the fluid obtained analysed for thiodiglycol. Papers by Vycudilik,[47] Drasch et al.,[48] Wils et al.,[49] Black and Read[50] and D'Agostino and Provost[51] should be consulted for details of the techniques used. The same estimation may be performed on blood and urine. The paper by Wils et al. is important, as it reports the results of investigations done on Iranian casualties.[49] Of the casualties, more than 80% had urine thiodiglycol levels above the 95% confidence limit for levels calculated for the control group. These investigations may be of some use in differentiating blistering produced by mustard from that produced by other agents, e.g. lewisite.

Temperature increases occur during the early stages of mustard poisoning and these plus the also typical early leukocytosis should not be taken uncritically as evidence of infection. Later the white cell count falls, the platelet count falls and finally the red cell count falls.

Culture of sputum and exudate from the eyes is important in order that appropriate antibiotic therapy may be given if infection supervenes. Infection of the chest is almost inevitable in a patient with extensive chemical lung damage and a very low white cell count. The dangers of infection are elaborated upon below.

MANAGEMENT OF CASES OF SULPHUR MUSTARD POISONING

Case management falls into two parts:

1. First aid measures
2. Therapeutic measures

First aid measures

These are of the greatest importance. Attendants should wear adequate protective clothing and respirators when dealing with contaminated casualties.

1. Patients should be removed from the source of contamination.
2. Areas of liquid contamination should be decontaminated using Fuller's earth in liberal quantities. Washing with organic solvents such as kerosene (paraffin) followed by soap and water is also valuable. Washing with organic solvents, if undertaken, should be continued for up to 30 min post-injury. The use of organic solvents was recommended by Vedder.[22] Chloramine solutions have also been extensively used.
3. Liquid contamination of the eyes should be immediately rinsed out using normal saline, if available, or any source of water.

Therapy and medical management

There is no specific therapy for sulphur mustard or nitrogen mustard poisoning. Perhaps because of this a considerable number of palliative approaches have been suggested. Some lessons have been learnt in this area from the extensive use of alkylating agents as antineoplastic drugs.

SKIN EFFECTS

For areas of erythema and minor blistering, bland lotions (e.g. calamine) have been suggested. Silver sulphadiazine (Flamazine) 1% cream was used in the management (1986) of Iranian mustard gas casualties.[42] This probably had value in reducing skin infection.

Dilute steroid preparations (Hydrocortisone Lotion) may be of symptomatic value in reducing irritation and itching. More powerful steroid preparations (beclomethasone dipropionate, i.e. 'Propaderm' cream) have also been used. Considerable symptomatic improvement was produced by the use of this preparation. Steroids have been suggested to delay healing and to enhance the likelihood of infection. No such ill-effects were observed in the Iranian casualties.

Severe pain and itching was reported by many of the Iranian mustard gas casualties. Therapy for pain ranged from paracetamol to morphine. It was found to be important to attempt to dissociate the pain from the panic exhibited by some patients, and diazepam in combination with a weak/mild analgesic proved, on several occasions, as effective as a potent analgesic. Very few patients were to require repeated doses of narcotic analgesics. Itching was troublesome in nearly all patients with extensive skin lesions, and prevented sleep. Antihistamines such as promethazine and dimethindine maleate proved effective. Carbamazepine was also used to great effect in one patient and allowed the use of narcotic analgesics to be stopped.

Willems (see above) reported a number of different patterns of management of skin lesions ranging from 'treating exposed' (at a burns unit) to treating by bathing and the use of wet dressings.[42] Skin lesions of Iranian patients treated in London, were, on the whole, treated exposed. Silver sulphadiazine cream was used if evidence of skin infection was obtained. Regular swabbing was undertaken.

An older remedy to control itching—benzyl alcohol, 100 parts; ethyl alcohol, 96 parts; glycerine, 4 parts—prepared as a paint might also be tried.

Large full-thickness burns will not heal satisfactorily without grafting. One Iranian casualty with severe and extensive skin damage was grafted and the grafts were found to take well. This is the only case the author has seen where skin grafting has been used in the management of sulphur mustard burns.

EYE EFFECTS

Early decontamination is the key. Attempts to decontaminate the eye when more than 5 min have passed after liquid contamination are likely to be valueless. It has been stated[52] that irrigation should:

> Be immediate; if it is delayed for longer than five minutes the eye may have been damaged and washing may only serve to increase the injury.

The concept of 'increasing the injury' presumably stems from the theory that any unabsorbed mustard may be spread by the washing to undamaged areas of the eye and subsequently cause damage there. Evidence for this is scanty, and if copious quantities of fluids are used in the washing process it is unlikely. For damaged eyes the following are suggested:

1. Saline irrigations.
2. Use of vaseline on follicular margins to prevent sticking.
3. If pain is severe, local anaesthetic drops, e.g. amethocaine hydrochloride (0.5%), should be used. Cocaine should be avoided, as it may produce sloughing of the corneal epithelium. To some extent all local anaesthetic preparations appear to damage the cornea. Some ophthalmologists advise the use of topical steroid preparations rather than of local anaesthetics. In the past steroids have been stated to be contraindicated in cases of mustard damage to the eyes. They were, however, used on a number of Iranian patients and no ill-effects were reported. Certainly, before they are used expert ophthalmological opinion should be sought. If eye pain is very severe, systemic narcotic analgesics should be used.
4. Chloramphenicol eye drops should be used to prevent infection. A number of different antibiotics were used in different centres by physicians managing Iranian chemical warfare casualties. These included: chloramphenicol, tetracycline, oxytetracycline, bacitracin and polymyxin B. No conclusions regarding the most effective drug could be drawn. There seems little reason to abandon the use of chloramphenicol eye drops.
5. Mydriatics such as hyoscine eye drops (0.25%) are useful in preventing sticking of the iris to the central area of the lens. In iritis mydriatic drops reduce pain due to spasm of the iris.
6. Dark glasses to alleviate photophobia.

Recently potassium ascorbate (10%) and sodium citrate (10%) drops have also been suggested. The ascorbate and citrate drops are to be given alternately every half-hour for all the waking day. The patient will therefore be receiving each preparation at hourly intervals. These drops may be discontinued once a stable epithelial covering has formed.[53]

In cases of severe eye damage an ophthalmological opinion *must be sought.*

Late corneal lesions are difficult to manage and blindness can occur. Contact lenses have proved very valuable for improving vision impaired by unevenness of the cornea.[38]

In all cases of mustard damage to the eyes, reassurance of severely frightened and often depressed patients is essential. During World War I great emphasis was placed upon encouraging those with eye damage to return to normal activity as soon as possible and not to become dependent upon dark glasses and eye drops. Prolonged eye irritation with profuse lacrimation and photophobia was encountered in one Iranian patient seen in London. Some 12 weeks post-exposure she was still unable to face bright lights, and tears poured almost continuously down her face. The cause of this very prolonged reaction is unknown.

As well as the above, a number of other methods have been proposed for managing mustard eye injuries.[54]

RESPIRATORY EFFECTS

There is no specific therapy for mustard injuries of the respiratory tract. Severe coughing may be eased with codeine linctus. Antibiotic cover is recommended, the antibiotic chosen not being one liable to induce further bone marrow depression. Acetylcysteine was used in some patients from the Iran–Iraq war as a mucolytic. Evidence of its efficacy is scanty.

In severe cases, respiratory failure may ensue. The management of such patients is complex and cannot be dealt with here. Advice from physicians and, if ventilation is necessary, anaesthetists *must* be sought.

BONE MARROW DEPRESSION

Bone marrow depression as a result of mustard poisoning is generally seen as therapeutically irreversible. If the aplastic anaemia produced is severe, granulocyte and platelet transfusions and later red cell transfusions should be considered. Bone marrow transplantation has also been suggested.

A number of drugs are known to stimulate the bone marrow (much of the evidence of this comes from studies of the effects of drugs on *normal* marrow). The value of such drugs in mustard poisoning is quite unknown. However, in view of the paucity of other approaches I list them:

1. Oxymethalone (a steroid)[55]
2. Lithium carbonate[56]
3. Glucan ($+ \beta$-1,3 polyglucose)[57]

More important than these drugs are the colony-stimulating factors which have recently become available. Granulocyte colony-stimulating factor and related factors should be considered in cases where bone marrow depression is marked.

It has been pointed out that cysteine can reduce the antitumour effects of alkylating agents.[26] In 1964, Connors et al. reported a reduction in toxicity of nitrogen mustards by pretreating rats with a variety of thiols.[58] Thiosulphate pretreatment (2 g kg^{-1} IP, i.e. maximum tolerated dose) produced an increase by a factor of 3.2 in the LD$_{50}$ of HN$_2$ if given 30 min before the mustard. Cysteine hydrochloride (L-cysteine hydrochloride, 1 g kg^{-1} IP, i.e. maximum tolerated dose) produced a five-fold increase in the LD$_{50}$ of HN$_2$ if given 30 min before the mustard. Table 5 is reproduced from the Connors paper.[58]

The work reported by Connors[58] followed work done at CDE by Callaway and Pearce reported in 1958.[59] They investigated the effects of thiosulphate/trisodium citrate mixtures (10 : 1, 2.75 g kg^{-1}, IP) on the toxicity of sulphur mustard in rats. The combination was referred to as Thiocit and it was demonstrated that:

> Thiocit afforded complete protection against greater than the median lethal dose of mustard gas whether given 10 minutes before or 10 minutes after mustard gas and raised the LD$_{50}$ of mustard gas approximately three times.

The use of Thiocit in conjunction with mustard gas therapy was suggested.

In 1986, Vojvodić reported a study of the protective effects of a number of compounds and combinations of compounds on the toxicity of nitrogen and sulphur mustards.[60] Protective indices similar to those obtained by Callaway were reported.

Work on the value of thiosulphate in the treatment of mustard gas poisoning has also been reported by Fasth.[61] Sodium thiosulphate has been recommended as a local treatment for accidentally extravasated doses of nitrogen mustards.[62]

Despite the above work, thiosulphate and other thiols have not achieved an established place in the treatment of mustard gas poisoning. Interestingly (see later) Russian sources have recommended intravenous infusion of 30% sodium thiosulphate in the treatment of mustard gas poisoning.

Attempts have been made to learn from work done to reduce the unwanted effects of anticancer therapy involving exposure to either radiation or high doses of alkylating agents. A useful review by Glover et al. should be consulted for details.[63] The compound WR-2721 has figured prominently in these studies.

Other measures which might be taken

If vomiting is a problem, then antiemetic drugs should be given. Phenothiazines would be a reasonable choice, though recent work has shown that blockers of 5HT$_3$ receptors may be of greater value. Work on such drugs is currently underway.

Haemodialysis and haemoperfusion have also been suggested and the latter recently used. Haemoperfusion was used in a few patients from the Iran–Iraq war. There is no sound theoretical basis for such therapy, as no active mustard has been

Table 5. Effect of thiosulphate and cysteine on LD_{50} of nitrogen mustards

Pretreatment 95%	Merophan (IP)			HN_2 (IP)			HN_2 (SC)		
	LD_{50} (mg kg^{-1})	Fiducial limits 95%	DRF	LD_{50} (mg kg^{-1})	Fiducial limits 95%	DRF	LD_{50} (mg kg^{-1})	Fiducial limits	DRF
None	3.67	3.24–4.16	1	1.28	1.08–1.51	1	2.06	1.74–2.43	1
Thiosulphate 2 g kg^{-1} IP, 30 min before	3.67	3.24–4.16	1	4.06	3.44–4.79	3.2	10.68	9.05–12.60	5.2
Cysteine 1 g kg^{-1} IP, 30 min before	15.24	13.65–16.71	4.2	6.33	5.37–7.46	4.9	10.68	9.39–12.14	5.2
Cysteine 1 g kg^{-1} + thiosulphate 2 g kg^{-1}	5.30	4.50–6.23	1.4	12.27	11.31–13.31	9.6	17.34	15.16–19.84	8.4

identified in blood taken from known mustard gas casualties. As a measure of last resort haemoperfusion might be justified, though the grave attendant risk of infection should be considered.

A range of general supportive measures were undertaken in Western centres treating casualties from the Iran–Iraq war. These included:

1. Use of H_2 antagonists to prevent stress ulceration.
2. Use of heparin in order to prevent deep venous thrombosis.
3. Use of vitamins C and B_{12} and folic acid.
4. Use of a single large dose of methylprednisolone (2 g) as general protection against tissue damage.

The above advice on management has been culled from a study of the Western literature of mustard gas poisoning. Measures recommended by eastern European sources differ substantially, in terms of drugs suggested, from the above. The following is taken from a Russian source.

For acute intoxication, intravenous infusion of:

- 40% glucose solution (20 ml; 1–2 daily)
- 30% sodium thiosulphate
- Calcium gluconate or chloride
- Cardiotonic drugs, e.g. camphor, caffeine
- Ascorbic acid (vitamin C)
- Thiamine (vitamin B_1)
- Pyridoxine (vitamin B_6)
- Blood transfusion

If leukopaenia and anaemia develop:

- Sodium nucleate, 0.5–1.0 g tds
- Methyl uracil, 1 g tds–qds
- Leucogen, 0.02 g tds
- Vitamin B_{12}, 0.01% solv, 1 ml, IV after 2–3 days

Note that sodium nucleate and leucogen are not recognized Western drugs.

PROGNOSIS FOR MUSTARD GAS CASUALTIES

As has already been pointed out, the great majority of mustard gas casualties survive. Resolution of specific problems can be difficult to predict but the following may provide a guide.

1. Eye lesions: most are resolved within 28 days of exposure.

2. Skin lesions: deep skin lesions may be expected to heal in up to 60 days. Superficial lesions heal in 14–21 days.
3. Upper respiratory tract lesions: it is very difficult to define a time course for complete recovery, as patients from the Iran–Iraq conflict were often discharged whilst still coughing and complaining of expectoration. Lung function tests on patients with purely upper respiratory tract lesions were usually normal on discharge. Patients with parenchymal damage often showed an abnormal pattern on lung function testing.

Leukopaenia is a common finding in mustard gas casualties. It is often comparatively minor and the white count recovers within 14 days. A marked fall in the white count is a serious event, and patients whose white counts fell to $< 200/mm^3$ did not survive despite artificial ventilation and intensive care. In all the cause of death was overwhelming infection and multiple organ failure.

LONG-TERM EFFECTS OF MUSTARD GAS POISONING

The long-term effects of mustard may be divided into three groups.

Psychological effects

The syndrome described earlier may persist for some time.

Local effects

These include:

- Permanent blindness
- Visual impairment
- Scarring of the skin
- Chronic bronchitis
- Bronchial stenosis
- Sensitivity to mustard gas

Carcinogenic effects

Sulphur mustard is a known human carcinogen.

The strongest evidence of induction of cancer by sulphur mustard comes from studies undertaken on mustard gas factory workers. The work of Wada *et al.*, Nishimoto *et al.* and Yanagida *et al.* should be consulted for details.[64–66] Exposures to mustard gas in these factories may have been considerable and prolonged. The study of British mustard gas workers revealed a clear increase in respiratory cancers.[67]

A more difficult question concerns the likelihood of developing cancer as a result of exposure to sulphur mustard on the battlefield. Here the evidence is suggestive but not absolutely clear-cut. The study by Norman[68] failed to demonstrate an increased risk of respiratory cancer in those exposed once to sulphur mustard. The study of Beebe[69] suggested that the incidence of lung cancer was higher in those exposed to mustard gas during World War I.

REFERENCES

1. West CJ (1920) The history of mustard gas. *Chem Metall Engin,* **22,** 541–554.
2. Meyer V (1886) Ueber Thiodiglycol verbindungen. *Berichte der Deutschen Chemische Gesellschaft (Berlin),* **XIX,** 3259–3265.
3. Prentiss AM (1937) *Chemicals in War.* New York: McGraw-Hill Book Company Inc.
4. Haldane JBS (1925) *Callinicus: A Defence of Chemical Warfare.* London: Kegan Paul, French, Tribner & Co. Ltd.
5. Lovatt Evans C (1970) *Biographical Memoirs of Fellows of the Royal Society,* Vol. 16.
6. Robinson JP (1971) The rise of CB weapons. In: *The Problem of Chemical and Biological Warfare.* New York: Stockholm International Peace Research Institute.
7. United Nations Security Council (1984) Report of the specialists appointed by the Secretary-General to investigate allegations by the Islamic Republic of Iran concerning the use of chemical weapons. United Nations Report S/16433.
8. United Nations Security Council (1986) Report of the mission despatched by the Secretary-General to investigate allegations of the use of chemical weapons in the conflict between the Islamic Republics of Iran and Iraq. United Nations Report S/17911.
9. United Nations Security Council (1987) Report of the mission despatched by the Secretary-General to investigate allegations of the use of chemical weapons in the conflict between the Islamic Republics of Iran and Iraq. United Nations Report S/18852.
10. Adair FE and Bagg HJ (1931) Experimental and clinical studies on the treatment of cancer by dichloroethylsulphide. *Ann Surg,* **93,** 190–199.
11. Pharmaceutical Society of Great Britain (1977) *Martindale. The Extra Pharmacopoeia,* (JEF Reynolds, ed.), 27th edn. London: The Pharmaceutical Press.
12. Ciszewka-Popiolek B, Czerny K, Swieca M *et al.* (1989) Der Einfluß des Präparats Psoriazin auf das morphologische und das histochemische Leberbild. (The effect of Psoriazin on the morphological and histochemical characteristics of the liver.) *Gegenbaurs Morphol Jahrb Leipzig,* **135,** 875–880.
13. Aasted A, Darre E and Wulf HC (1987) Mustard gas: clinical, toxicological and mutagenic aspects based on modern experience. *Ann Plast Surg,* **19,** 330–333.
14. Cullumbine H (1947) The mode of penetration of the skin by mustard gas. *Br J Dermatol,* **58,** 291–294.
15. Nagy JM, Golumbic C, Stein WH *et al.* (1946) The penetration of vapours into human skin. *J Gen Physiol,* **29,** 441–469.
16. Renshaw B (1946) Mechanisms in production of cutaneous injuries by sulfur and nitrogen mustards. In: *Chemical Warfare Agents and Related Chemical Problems,* Vol. 1, pp. 479–518. Washington DC: US Office of Scientific Research and Development, National Defense Research Committee.
17. Papirmeister B, Gross CL, Petrali JP *et al.* (1984) Pathology produced by sulfur mustard in human skin grafts on athymic nude mice. I. Gross and light microscopic changes. *J Toxicol Cutan Ocul Toxicol,* **3,** 371–391.
18. Papirmeister B, Gross CL, Petrali JP *et al.* (1984) Pathology produced by sulfur mustard

in human skin grafts on athymic nude mice. II. Ultrastructural changes. *J Toxicol Cutan Ocul Toxicol*, **3**, 393–408.

19. Cameron GR, Gaddum JH and Short RHD (1946) The absorption of war gases by the nose. *J Pathol*, **58**, 449–497.

20. Black RM, Brewster K, Clarke RJ *et al.* (1993) Metabolism of thiodiglycol (2,2′-thiobis-ethanol): isolation and identification of urinary metabolites following intraperitoneal administration to rat. *Xenobiotica*, **23**, 473–481.

21. Davison C, Rozman RS and Smith PK (1961) Metabolism of bis-β-chlorethyl sulfide (sulphur mustard gas). *Biochem Pharmacol*, **7**, 65–74.

22. Vedder EB (1925) *The Medical Aspects of Chemical Warfare*. Baltimore: Williams and Wilkins Co.

23. NATO (1985) *Handbook on the Medical Aspects of NBC Defensive Operations*. AMedP-6. Part III. Chemical.

24. Zaniboni A, Simoncini E, Marpicati P *et al.* (1988) Severe delayed neurotoxicity after accidental high-dose nitrogen mustard. *Am J Hematol*, **27**, 304.

25. Bethlenfalvay NC and Bergin JJ (1972) Severe cerebral toxicity after intravenous nitrogen mustard therapy. *Cancer*, **29**, 366–369.

26. Bowman WC, Bowman A and Bowman A (1986) *Dictionary of Pharmacology*. Oxford: Blackwell Scientific.

27. Goodman L and Gilman A (eds) (1980) *The Pharmacologic Basis of Therapeutics*. New York, London: Macmillan, Baillière Tindall.

28. Fox M and Scott D (1980) The genetic toxicology of nitrogen and sulphur mustard. *Mutat Res*, **75**, 131–168.

29. Juarez-Salinas H, Sims JL and Jacobson MK (1979) Poly(ADP-ribose) levels in carcinogen treated cells. *Nature*, **282**, 740–741.

30. Meier HL, Gross CL and Papirmeister B (1987) 2,2′-Dichlorodiethyl sulfide (sulfur mustard) decreases NAD^+ levels in human leukocytes. *Toxicol Lett*, **39**, 109–122.

31. Dixon M and Needham DM (1946) Biochemical research on chemical warfare agents. *Nature*, **158**, 432–438.

32. Miskin R and Reich E (1980) Plasminogen activator: induction of synthesis by DNA damage. *Cell*, **19**, 217–224.

33. McAdams AJ (1956) A study of mustard vesication. *J Invest Dermatol*, **26**, 317–326.

34. Hunt C and Phillips S (1949) Acute pharmacology of methyl bis(2-chloroethyl)amine (NH_2). *J Pharmacol Exp Ther*, **95**, 131–144.

35. Ireland MM (1926) Medical aspects of gas warfare. *The Medical Department of the United States in the World War*, Vol. XIV. Washington DC.

36. Vogt RF, Dannenberg AM, Schofield BH *et al.* (1984) Pathogenesis of skin lesions caused by sulphur mustard. *Fundam Appl Toxicol*, **4**, S71–S83.

37. Sulzberger MC, Baer RI, Kanof A *et al.* (1947) Skin sensitization to vesicant agents of chemical warfare. *J Invest Dermatol*, **8**, 365–393.

38. Mann I, Pirie A and Pullinger BD (1948) An experimental and clinical study of the reaction of the anterior segment of the eye in chemical injury, with special reference to chemical warfare agents. *Br J Ophthalmol*, Suppl. XII, 1–171.

39. Warthin AS and Weller CV (1918) The pathology of skin lesions produced by mustard gas (dichloroethylsulphide). *J Lab Clin Med*, **3**, 447–486.

40. Friendenwald JS, Scholz RO, Snell A *et al.* (1948) Studies on the physiology, bio-chemistry and cytopathology of the cornea in relation to injury by mustard gas and allied toxic agents. I. Introduction and outline. *Bull Johns Hopkins Hospital*, No. 2, 81–101.

41. Pappenheimer AM and Vance M (1920) The delayed action of mustard gas and lewisite. *J Exp Med*, **31**, 71–94.

42. Willems JL (1989) Clinical management of mustard gas casualties. *Ann Med Militaries Belgicae*, **3** (Suppl.), 1–61.

43. Sulzberger MB and Katz JH (1943) The absence of skin irritants in the contents of vesicles. *US Navy Med Bull*, **43**, 1258–1262.
44. Stockholm International Peace Research Institute (1971) *The Problem of Chemical and Biological Warfare*. New York: Stockholm International Peace Research Institute.
45. Norris K (1986) Personal communication.
46. Lefebure V (1921) *The Riddle of the Rhine*. London: W. Collins Sons & Co.
47. Vycudilik W (1985) Detection of mustard gas bis(2-chloroethyl)-sulfide in urine. *Forensic Sci Int*, **28**, 131–136.
48. Drasch G, Kretschmet E, Kauert E *et al.* (1987) Concentrations of mustard gas (bis(e-chloroethyl)sulfide) in the tissues of a victim of a vesicant exposure. *J Forensic Sci*, **32**, 1788–1793.
49. Wils ERJ, Hulst AG and van Laar J (1988) Analysis of thiodiglycol in urine of victims of an alleged attack with mustard gas, part II. *J Anal Toxicol*, **12**, 15–19.
50. Black RM and Read RW (1988) Detection of trace levels of thiodiglycol in blood, plasma and urine using gas chromatography–electron capture negative-ion chemical ionisation mass spectrometry. *J Chromatogr*, **449**, 261–270.
51. D'Agostino PA and Provost LR (1988) Gas chromatographic retention indices of sulfur vesicants and related compounds. *J Chromatogr*, **436**, 399–411.
52. Ministry of Defence (1987) *Medical Manual of Defence Against Chemical Agents*. Ministry of Defence D/Med(F & S)(2)/10/1/1. London: HMSO.
53. Wright P (1990) Personal communication.
54. Foster J (1939) Ophthalmic injuries from mustard gas (D.E.S.). *Br Med J*, **2**, 1181–1183.
55. Pharmaceutical Society of Great Britain (1989) *Martindale. The Extra Pharmacopoeia* (JEF Reynolds, ed.), 29th edn. London: The Pharmaceutical Press.
56. Lyman GH, Williams CC and Preston D (1980) The use of lithium carbonate to reduce infection and leukopenia during systemic chemotherapy. *N Engl J Med*, **302**, 257–260.
57. Di Luzio NR (1983) Immunopharmacology of glucan: a broad spectrum enhancer of host defense mechanisms. *Trends Pharmacol Sci*, **4**, 344–347.
58. Connors TA, Jeny A and Jones M (1964) Reduction of the toxicity of 'radiomimetic' alkylating agents in rats by thiol pretreatment—III. The mechanism of the protective action of thiosulphate. *Biochem Pharmacol*, **13**, 1545–1550.
59. Callaway S and Pearce KA (1958) Protection against systemic poisoning by mustard gas, (di(2-chloroethyl) sulphide), by sodium thiosulphate and thiocit in the albino rat. *Br J Pharmacol*, **13**, 395–398.
60. Vojvodić V, Milosavljević Z, Bošković B *et al.* (1985) The protective effect of different drugs in rats poisoned by sulfur and nitrogen mustards. *Fundam Appl Toxicol*, **5**, S160–S168.
61. Fasth A and Sörbo B (1973) Protective effect of thiosulfate and metabolic thiosulfate precursors against toxicity of nitrogen mustard (HN$_2$). *Biochem Pharmacol*, **22**, 1337–1351.
62. Dorr RT, Soble M and Alberts DS (1988) Efficacy of sodium thiosulfate as a local antidote to mechlorethamine skin toxicity in the mouse. *Cancer Chemother Pharmacol*, **22**, 299–302.
63. Glover D, Fox KR, Weiler C *et al.* (1988) Clinical trials of WR-2721 prior to alkylating agent chemotherapy and radiotherapy. *Pharmacol Ther*, **39**, 3–7.
64. Wada S, Miyanishi M, Nishimoto Y *et al.* (1968) Mustard gas as a cause of respiratory neoplasia in man. *Lancet*, **i**, 1161–1163.
65. Nishimoto Y, Yamakido M, Ishioka S *et al.* (1988) Epidemiological status of lung cancer in Japanese mustard gas workers. In: *Unusual Occurrences as Clues to Cancer Aetiology* (RW Miller *et al.*, eds), pp. 95–101. Tokyo: Japan Scientific Society Press, Taylor & Francis.
66. Yanagida J, Hozawa S, Ishioka S *et al.* (1988) Somatic mutation in peripheral

lymphocytes of former workers at the Okunojima poison gas factory. *Jpn J Cancer Res*, **79**, 1276–1283.

67. Easton DF, Peto J and Doll R (1988) Cancers of the respiratory tract in mustard gas workers. *Br J Ind Med*, **45**, 652–659.
68. Norman JE (1975) Lung cancer mortality in World War I veterans with mustard-gas injury: 1919–1965. *J Natl Cancer Inst*, **54**, 311–317.
69. Beebe GW (1960) Lung cancer in World War I veterans: possible relation to mustard gas injury and 1918 influenza epidemic. *J Natl Cancer Inst*, **5**, 1231–1251.

7

ORGANIC ARSENICALS

A number of organic arsenicals have been developed for use as chemical warfare agents, the majority during World War I. Of these, by far the most important is lewisite, isolated in pure form by Lee Lewis in 1918 (Table 1). Lewisite was developed in an attempt to provide a highly toxic, non-persistent, quick-acting vesicant compound. Mustard gas had been used on a large scale during World War I but its long persistence made it difficult for attacks to be launched on contaminated ground. Ethyldichlorarsine and diphenylchlorarsine were used by German troops, though they were not as effective as had been expected.

LEWISITE

Lewisite (2-chlorovinyldichloroarsine) was first synthesized in bulk in the USA and according to Prentiss[1] the first shipment was on its way to Europe when the 1918 armistice was agreed: this shipment was apparently destroyed at sea. As pointed out in Chapter 1, lewisite rapidly acquired a remarkable reputation as the 'Dew of Death', though there remains no proof of it having been used in war.

Lewisite is an odorless, colorless oily liquid of structural formula $ClCH=CHAsCl_2$ (Table 2). Lewisite is said to darken on standing, and technical preparations are often blue-black to black in color and are said to smell of geraniums. Lewisite, which is not soluble in water to any appreciable extent, nevertheless hydrolyzes rapidly when mixed with water and is rapidly hydrolyzed by

Table 1. Organic arsenicals of chemical warfare importance

Chemical name	Other names
2-Chlorovinyldichlorarsine	Lewisite
Ethyldichlorarsine	Dick
Methylarsine	Methyl dick
Phenyldichlorarsine	Sneeze Gas
Diphenylchlorarsine	DA, Clark 1
Diphenylcyanarsine	DC, Clark 2
Diphenylaminechlorarsine	DM, Adamsite

Table 2 Physical properties of lewisite

Boiling point	190°C
Melting point	−13°C
Vapor pressure	at 0°C, 0.087 mmHg
	at 20°C, 0.395 mmHg

alkaline aqueous solutions such as sodium hypochlorite solution. The rapid hydrolysis of lewisite by water and especially by alkalis was seen to be advantageous to troops using the compound as a weapon, but this property can nevertheless be a disadvantage in that it is unlikely that lewisite would be an effective weapon under wet conditions. Such conditions would render maintenance of effective field difficult. Prentiss[1] gave the persistence of lewisite at 20°C as 9.6 times that of water, whereas the persistence of sulfur mustard is 67 times that of water at the same temperature. The freezing point of lewisite is −18°C and thus no special preparations, of the type required with mustard, are needed for use under most winter conditions.

ABSORPTION

Lewisite is rapidly absorbed through the skin and mucous membranes. The distribution of lewisite has been assumed to follow that of other arsenicals, but this is probably not the case. The distribution of organomercurials and organotins is different from that of the inorganic salts of those metals, and Inns et al.[2] found that in rabbits, at doses of equal lethal toxicity, tissue levels of arsenic were much higher with sodium arsenite than with lewisite. There was a notable exception, namely the lungs, where tissue levels were slightly higher with lewisite. Bearing in mind that the intravenous lethal dose of lewisite is, on an arsenic content basis, much lower than that of sodium arsenite, the arsenic of lewisite clearly preferentially distributes to the lung. Inns et al.[2] attributed the differences that they observed in toxic effects of lewisite and inorganic arsenic salts to differences in disposition. In fact, comparatively little is known of the biotransformation of organic arsenicals,[3] but it is known that trivalent arsenicals are converted to pentavalent derivatives and that these occur in the urine. Pentavalent arsenicals are less toxic than compounds of trivalent arsenic.

MODE OF EXPOSURE

As lewisite is a liquid, it may be disseminated by shells, bombs or rockets or sprayed from aircraft. Lewisite can be mixed with sulfur mustard, a course which depresses the freezing point and renders sulfur mustard usable over a wider range of temperatures.

Individuals may be contaminated by contact with liquid or by inhalation of the vapor.

Table 3 Acute toxicity of lewisite

Species	Route	LD_{50} (mg kg^{-1}) (95% CL if available)	Reference
Rat	PO	50	US Army[5]
Rat	PC	24	Cited in Maynard[4]
Rabbit	IV	0.5	Cited in Maynard[4]
Rabbit	IV	1.8 (1.6–2.1)	Inns *et al.*[2]
Rabbit	PC	6	Cited in Maynard[4]
Rabbit	PC	5.3 (3.5–8.5)	Inns and Rice[6]
Guinea pig	PC	12	Cited in Maynard[4]
Dog	PC	15	Cited in Maynard[4]

PC, percutaneous; IV, intravenous; PO, oral.

TOXICOLOGY

Acute toxicity figures for humans are not known but a lowest lethal concentration over 30 min of 6 ppm was quoted by Maynard.[4] The LD_{50} has been measured in a number of species (Table 3), while LCt_{50}s in a variety of species vary from 500 to 1500 mg min m^{-3}.[7] The efficacy of lewisite, like that of mustard, depends upon its vesicant properties but lewisite is also a lethal chemical weapon. About 30 drops (2.6 g), applied to the skin and not washed off or otherwise decontaminated, would be expected to be fatal to an average man.

MODE OF ACTION

Arsenic, like most heavy metals, binds to a wide range of compounds, including macromolecules such as proteins, which contain sulfhydryl groups.[8] Many of the effects of lewisite are thought to be due to binding to dihydrolipoic acid, a component of the pyruvate dehydrogenase complex.[9–11] This prevents formation of acetyl coenzyme A from pyruvate. Peters demonstrated 50% inhibition of the activity of the pyruvate dehydrogenase system with 15×10^{-6} M sodium arsenite, and observed that in animals treated with sodium arsenite, blood levels of pyruvate rose.

PATHOLOGY

SKIN

The pathological effects of lewisite have been less studied than those of other vesicants, particularly sulfur mustard. Ireland[12] studied the progression of the lesion after the application of lewisite to the skin of horses. Five hours after exposure, marked edema of the skin was noted, extending into the dermis with separation of collagen fibers. More deeply placed blood vessels were surrounded by collections of polymorphs. By 24 h, there was thinning of the epidermis with nuclear pyknosis. The dermis was edematous and there were collections of fluid at the epidermal–dermal junction. At 48 h, there was a definite margin to the lesion and some repair was noted; damaged areas were heavily pigmented. In comparison with mustard, lewisite produced epidermal necrosis earlier, with more extensive edema and inflammation, and more vascular thrombosis. On the other hand, repair with lewisite appeared to start earlier than with mustard. Recent work by King et al.[13] suggested that in lewisite-treated isolated perfused porcine skin flaps, epidermal–dermal separation was localized in the lamina lucida. It was hypothesized by these workers that chemical modification of the glycoprotein adhesive, laminin, was responsible.

Lewisite is markedly vesicant when applied to human skin, but vesication has not been observed in animals so far studied.

RESPIRATORY TRACT

The main effect of lewisite on the upper respiratory tract is to produce necrosis of the epithelium, which is accompanied by the formation of a false diphtheria-type membrane which consists of sloughed epithelial cells together with inflammatory cells and mucus. The membrane may become detached and cause bronchial obstruction. Widespread edema and congestion of the lungs occurs, and they may acquire a grayish-red to purple hue. Areas of atelectasis and secondary emphysema are common. Secondary bronchopneumonia is common and a frequent cause of death.[14]

Marked edema of mediastinal structures, including the pericardium, is seen.

EYE

Detailed pathological descriptions of the effects of lewisite on the eye are not available.

SYSTEMIC PATHOLOGICAL EFFECTS

In the studies of Inns et al.[2,15] with lewisite injected intravenously into rabbits, changes in the lungs, including hemorrhage and edema, with lymphocytic infiltration, were seen. Damage was found in the biliary tree, including epithelial necrosis in the gall bladder. Inns and Rice,[6] in a study in which lewisite was applied to the skin, observed focal hepatocyte degeneration and transmural necrosis of the gall bladder. Small bile duct proliferation and early portal tract fibrosis was seen and there was focal mucosal necrosis in the duodenum; however, lung changes of the type seen with intravenous lewisite were not observed. Taken together, these data show clearly that the toxicity of lewisite is neither qualitatively nor quantitatively just that of the arsenic that it contains (see above).

Symptoms and clinical signs

Because lewisite has not been used in warfare, descriptions are mainly derived from accidental exposure, or else clinical signs in humans have been inferred from observations in animals.

Immediately after exposure, there is eye irritation, and coughing, sneezing, salivation and lacrimation rapidly follow. Contamination of the skin causes erythema at concentrations of 0.05–0.01 mg/cm^{-2},[15] with vesication after a few hours. Pain in the skin and eyes is immediate, a major point of difference from sulfur mustard. The effects in the eye and skin reach their greatest at 4–8 h post-exposure. The patient is seriously incapacitated, breathing with difficulty and unable to see. In severe cases pulmonary edema follows and the patient may die of respiratory failure. Decontamination is very important.[16] In cases where skin contamination is extensive, there may be liver necrosis and the absorption of arsenic may be sufficient to cause death.

The eye lesions produced by lewisite are particularly serious: blindness will follow contamination of the eye with liquid lewisite unless decontamination is very prompt. It is possible to infer from animal experiments undertaken in the USA during World War II that exposure of the eye to liquid or vapor would produce blepharospasm and irritation. Severe ocular lesions can be produced by doses as low as 0.1 mg or exposure to the saturated vapor for 8 s at 23°C. The action on the eye is to produce rapid necrosis of the anterior parts of that organ.[17]

It has been said that absorption of lewisite in food would be expected to give rise to the symptoms and signs of arsenical poisoning. These include severe stomach pain, vomiting, watery diarrhea, numbness and tingling, particularly in the feet, thirst and muscular cramps. Neuropathy, nephritis with proteinuria and/or encephalopathy may follow acute arsenical poisoning. Intravascular hemolysis and hemolytic anemia may occur, with, in extreme cases, renal failure.[18] Nevertheless, the view that lewisite is simply arsenic poisoning is clearly false, and parenteral lewisite differs from inorganic arsenic in significant respects (see above): the same may be true of lewisite by the oral route.

First-hand accounts of the effects of exposure to lewisite under battlefield conditions are, as has already been noted, unavailable. However, the effects of phenyldichlorarsine, a related arsenical vesicant, have been described by Hunter.[19] Hunter's description is reproduced from *The Diseases of Occupations* by permission of the publishers (Hodder and Stoughton, London).

KT-T, a man of 39 ... had been put to work on 21 August 1940 on a bulk supply of liquid arsenical vesicant containing phenyldichlorarsine. By mistake he was wearing rubber gloves which had been condemned as too thin to give adequate protection. He had spilled some of the liquid over the back of his right hand glove, had wiped the glove and, thinking it was impervious to the liquid, had gone on wearing it for two hours longer. That night the dorsum of the right hand was red and painful. By the next morning it was severely blistered from the middle of the fingers to three inches above the wrist. The palm was unaffected. His wife, who handled a towel soiled by the blister fluid, suffered later from minor burns to the skin of her hands. Two days later he had to go to bed because of severe diarrhoea, vomiting and slight jaundice. For about a week he vomited up to four times a day and for twelve days he had diarrhoea in which he passed on an average six fluid stools daily without blood. The skin of the hand was healed by the tenth day. The jaundice disappeared after three weeks. Minor attacks of diarrhoea had occurred subsequently over a period of three years.

A number of interesting lessons can be drawn from this account.

Phenyldichlorarsine is a less severe vesicant than lewisite, though Prentiss described its vesicant actions as 'not inconsiderable'. The capacity of the arsenical compound to penetrate a possibly thin rubber glove is clear and should be borne in mind by those who are decontaminating casualties. The systemic effects of absorbed arsenic are clearly reported.

That the patient's wife should have been affected by contact with a towel contaminated with blister fluid is puzzling. In Chapter 6 the observation that blister fluid from blisters produced by both sulfur mustard and lewisite was not an irritant was reported. It may be that the towel was contaminated directly with phenyl-dichlorarsine.

Phenyldichlorarsine was used on a large scale during World War I. It was used as a compound capable of penetrating the respirators then available and also capable of producing severe irritation of the respiratory tract. It was apparently a very effective chemical weapon.

Therapy

FIRST AID

The casualty must be removed from the source of contamination; rescue workers must be protected against liquid lewisite by protective clothing, gloves and boots and against the vapour by respirators. Because of the danger to both the casualty and the attendants, it is essential that standard drills be followed when decontaminating a casualty whose protective clothing is contaminated with lewisite. Fuller's earth is an effective decontaminant; dilute solutions of bleach would also be effective.

SPECIFIC THERAPY

Unlike vesicants of the mustard group, highly effective specific therapy is available for poisoning with organic arsenicals. Since World War II, dimercaprol (British Anti-Lewisite, BAL, 2,3-dimercaptopropanol) has been the standard treatment for poisoning by arsenic compounds, including lewisite and other organic arsenicals. Dimercaprol binds to lewisite as follow:

$$\begin{array}{c} CH_2SH \\ | \\ CHSH \\ | \\ CH_2OH \end{array} + \begin{array}{c} Cl \\ \diagdown \\ \diagup \\ Cl \end{array} AsCH{=}CHCl \rightarrow \begin{array}{c} CH_2S \\ | \diagdown \\ CHS \diagup \\ | \\ CH_2OH \end{array} AsCH{=}CHCl + 2HCl$$

In animal studies, dimercaprol was able to protect against the effects of lewisite and reverse the enzyme inhibition produced by it. Dimercaprol was originally developed for parenteral use against systemic lewisite poisoning, and it was also available as an ointment for use against skin burns. However, dimercaprol has major disadvantages as an antidote. When used for systemic arsenic poisoning the dose of dimercaprol is limited by toxicity and the drug has to be given by intramuscular injection. Dimercaprol is dissolved in peanut oil and benzyl benzoate and injections are painful.[20,21] Furthermore, the material cannot be given intravenously, denying the possibilities of a loading dose.

A number of different dosing regimes have been recommended; thus JSP 312[22] suggests:

- 2.5 mg kg^{-1} 4-hourly for four doses; then
- 2.5 mg kg^{-1} twice daily.

Martindale[23] gives the following regime:

- Day 1: 400–800 mg IM in divided doses
- Days 2 and 3: 200–400 mg IM in divided doses
- Days 4–12: 100–200 mg IM in divided doses

Within this range the dose is determined by body weight and the severity of symptoms. Administration should be by deep intramuscular injection using multiple injection sites. Intramuscular dimercaprol may produce alarming reactions. Pain at the injection site may last for up to 24 h, while systemic reactions include increased blood pressure and tachycardia, nausea and vomiting, headache and feelings of constriction of the chest. Conjunctivitis, lacrimation, rhinorrhea, sweating, anxiety and agitation have also been reported. These effects pass in a few hours. Klaassen[2] emphasized the need to maintain a high plasma level of the drug so that the rapidly excreted 2:1 complex of dimercaprol–arsenic should predominate over the 1:1 complex, which is more slowly excreted.

Skin contamination should be treated with dimercaprol ointment. Eye contamination can be treated by application of dimercaprol (5–10% in vegetable oil) into the conjunctival sac. This should be performed as a matter of urgency. The eye drops produce pain on instillation in this way.

Two water-soluble analogs of dimercaprol have been studied as lewisite antidotes, *meso*-2,3-dimercaptosuccinic acid (DMSA) and 2,3-dimercapto-1-propanesulfonic acid (DMPS). Their structures are shown on p. 182.

These drugs circumvent two major disadvantages of dimercaprol discussed above, namely the need for intramuscular injection and the limitation of dose by toxicity. DMSA and DMPS are about 20 and 10 times less toxic than dimercaprol in the mouse[24] and can be given orally. Inns *et al.*[15] showed that, in rabbits poisoned with intravenous lewisite, dimercaprol, DMPS and DMSA were, on a molar basis, equieffective, but emphasized the limitations in dosage conferred by the toxicity of

DMSA	DMPS
COOH	CH_2SH
$\mid$	$\mid$
CHSH	CHSH
$\mid$	$\mid$
CHSH	$CH_2SO_3^- \ Na^+$
$\mid$	
COOH	

dimercaprol. Studying the antidotal efficacy of dimercaprol, DMSA and DMPS against lewisite applied percutaneously to rabbits, Inns and Rice[6] concluded that, at equimolar doses (40 μmol 1^{-1}), there was little difference between the efficacy of dimercaprol, DMPS and DMSA; however, the low toxicity of DMPS and DMSA enabled the use of high doses of antidotes which produced improved survival, while dimercaprol at these molar doses would have been toxic. Protection ratios (LD_{50} with treatment/LD_{50} without treatment) were 13 and 16.9 respectively for DMPS and DMSA at the higher dose of 160 μmol kg^{-1} IM. Hepatocellular damage (see above) appeared to be reduced by chelation therapy. Despite the evidence that at equimolar doses the three chelators are more or less equieffective, the two more novel drugs may have advantages other than just their low toxicity. Thus Aposhian et al.[24] showed that dimercaprol was the least effective of the three in reversing arsenite inhibition of the pyruvate dehydrogenase complex in the kidneys of mice or in a mouse kidney system in vitro. Another possible advantage of DMPS and DMSA over dimercaprol is that the last-named drug increased the arsenic content of brains of rabbits poisoned with sodium arsenite, whereas the first two do not;[24] however, this observation should be treated with some circumspection, as it is possible that the arsenic was not biologically active.

DMPS and DMSA applied to the skin would probably be of value in lewisite-induced vesication. However, the disadvantages of dimercaprol largely relate to systemic treatment and the water-soluble analogs are unlikely to be better than dimercaprol ointment.

Other measures that may prove necessary include antibiotics to treat broncho-pneumonia; the prophylactic use of antibiotics is controversial.

OTHER ORGANIC ARSENICALS

Ethyl-, methyl- and phenyldichlorarsine are known as the Dicks; more specifically, ethyldichlorarsine is dick and methyldichloarsine is methyl dick. They are vesicants similar to lewisite, and dichlorarsine was used by the Germans in World War I to a limited extent. Phenyldichlorarsine was used in some percutaneous studies by Aposhian et al;[24] these suggested that DMPS and DMSA would be useful in prophylaxis against skin burns.

Diphenylchlorarsine, diphenylcyanarsine and diphenylaminechlorarsine are irritants.

REFERENCES

1. Prentiss AM (1937) *Chemicals in War.* McGraw-Hill Book Company: New York.
2. Inns RH, Bright JE and Marrs TC (1988) Comparative acute systemic toxicity of sodium arsenite and dichloro(2-chlorovinyl)arsine in rabbits. *Toxicology*, **51**, 213–222.
3. Klaassen CD (1985) Heavy metals and heavy metal antagonists. In: *Goodman and Gilman's The Pharmacological Basis of Therapeutics* (AG Gilman, LS Goodman, TW Rall and F Murad, eds), 7th edn, pp. 1605–1627. New York: Macmillan.
4. Maynard RL (1989) A review of chemical warfare agents. CDE Technical Paper, 2nd edn. Porton Down: CDE.
5. US Army (1974) *Chemical Data Sheets*, Vol. I. Report EO-SR-74001, pp. 65–72. Edgewood Arsenal, Maryland. Development and Engineering Directorate.
6. Inns RH and Rice P (1993) Efficacy of dimercapto chelating agents for the treatment of poisoning by percutaneously applied dichloro(2-chlorovinyl)arsine in rabbits. *Human Exp Toxicol*, **12**, 241–246.
7. Goldman M and Dacre JC (1989) Lewisite: its chemistry, toxicology and biological effects. *Rev Environ Contam Toxicol*, **110**, 75–115.
8. Ehrlich P (1909) Über den jetzigen Stand der Chemotherapie. *Ber Deutsch Chem. Ges.*, **42**, 17.
9. Peters R (1945) British anti-lewisite (BAL). *Nature*, **156**, 616.
10. Peters R (1948) Development and theoretical significance of British Anti-Lewisite (BAL). *Br Med Bull*, **5**, 313.
11. Peters R (1953) Significance of biochemical lesions in the pyruvate oxidase system. *Br Med Bull*, **9**, 116.
12. Ireland MW (1926) Medical aspects of chemical warfare. In: *The Medical Department of the US Army in World War I*, Vol. XIV. Washington: Government Printing Office.
13. King JR, Peters BP and Monteiro-Riviere NA (1994) Laminin in the cutaneous basement membrane as a potential target in lewisite vesication. *Toxicol Appl Pharmacol*, **126**, 164–173.
14. Vedder EB (1926) *The Medical Aspects of Chemical Warfare.* Baltimore: Williams and Wilkins.
15. Inns RH, Rice P, Bright JE and Marrs TC (1990) Evaluation of the efficacy of dimercapto chelating agents for the treatment of systemic organic arsenic poisoning in rabbits. *Human Exp Toxicol*, **9**, 215–220.
16. Ottinger RS, Blumenthal JL, Dal Porto DF *et al.* (1973) *Recommended methods of reduction, neutralization, recovery, or disposal of hazardous wastes.* Vol. VII. *Propellants, explosives, chemical warfare.* Report EPA-670/2-73-052-8. Washington DC: US Environmental Protection Agency.
17. Friedenwald JS and Hughes WF (1948) The effects of toxic chemical agents on the eyes and their treatment. In: *Advances in Military Medicine*, Vol II. Boston: Little, Brown and Co.
18. Stewart CE and Sullivan JB (1992) Military munitions and antipersonnel agents. In: *Hazardous Materials Toxicology* (JB Sullivan and GR Krieger, eds), pp. 986–1026. Baltimore: Williams and Wilkins.
19. Hunter D (1978) *The Diseases of Occupations*, 6th edn, pp. 368–369. London: Hodder and Stoughton.
20. Sulzberger MB, Boer RL and Kanof A (1946) Clinical uses of 2,3-dimercaptopropanol

(BAL) III. Studies on the toxicity of BAL on percutaneous and parenteral administrations. *J Clin Invest*, **25**, 474–479.

21. Modell W, Gould H and Cattell M (1946) Clinical uses of 2,3-dimercapto-propanol (BAL). IV Pharmacologic observations on BAL by intramuscular injection in man. *J Clin Invest*, **25**, 480–487.
22. JSP 312 (1972) *Medical Manual of Defence against Chemical Agents*. London: HMSO.
23. Martindale (1993) *The Extra Pharmacopoeia*, 30th edn (JEF Reynolds, ed.). London: Pharmaceutical Press.
24. Aposhian HV, Carter CD, Hoover TD *et al.* (1984) DMSA, DMPS and DMPA as arsenic antidotes. *Fundam Appl Toxicol*, **4**, S58–S70.

8

PHOSGENE

Phosgene is a colourless gas first prepared by John Davy in 1812. It was developed as a chemical weapon by German workers during World War I (WWI) and was first used, against British troops, near Ypres on 19 December 1915. Four thousand cylinders of phosgene (88 tons) were released, causing 1069 casualties and 120 deaths. By 1915, the Allied forces had also been experimenting with phosgene and the gas was later used on a substantial scale by both sides. Phosgene had been used as an intermediate in the dye industry for many years and was being produced, on a large scale, in Germany before WWI. The effect of the dominance of the German dye industry on the development of chemical warfare has been commented on by Lefebure[1] and in Chapter 1.

Phosgene accounted for some 85% of all deaths attributed to chemical weapons during WWI.[2] Despite this, its efficacy as a chemical warfare agent was probably less than that of mustard gas. Phosgene acts by damaging the lungs and producing pulmonary oedema: it was thus classified, amongst other lung-damaging agents, with chloropicrin, trichloromethyl chloroformate and disulphur decafluoride. The lethality of phosgene and other lung-damaging agents led to an intensive search for more effective agents during WWI: an excellent account has been provided by Prentiss.[3]

CHEMICAL AND PHYSICAL PROPERTIES OF PHOSGENE

Phosgene is, at ordinary temperatures and pressures, a colourless gas with a suffocating smell said to be reminiscent of mouldy hay. Its physical properties are shown in Table 1.

Table 1. Physical properties of phosgene

Formula	$COCl_2$
Melting point	$-118°C$
Boiling point	$8.2°C$
MW	99
Vapour pressure at 20°C	1215 mmHg
Vapour density	3.5

Early studies of the reaction between phosgene and water suggested that the hydrolysis of phosgene proceeded slowly.[4] This is untrue: Potts *et al.*[5] showed that hydrolysis occurred rapidly with the production of hydrochloric acid:

$$COCl_2 + H_2O \rightarrow CO_2 + 2HCl$$

The rapidity of hydrolysis was also noted by Prentiss, who pointed out that phosgene could not be used successfully in wet weather.[3] Production of hydrochloric acid in shells containing phosgene and some water was also identified as a problem by Prentiss.

It should be noted that, though the boiling point of phosgene (8.2°C) is below normal summer temperatures, the rate of evaporation of liquid phosgene is slow compared with that of chlorine (BP: −33.6°C) and to produce adequately lethal gas clouds chlorine was almost always mixed with phosgene: this was in fact done during the first phosgene attack referred to above.

LIKELY MODE OF EXPOSURE TO PHOSGENE

Phosgene can be disseminated by aircraft, from pressurized containers and by bombs and shells. The gas is rapidly dispersed by the wind, though, as it is heavier than air, it tends to accumulate in low-lying areas and dangerous concentrations may occur in cellars and trenches. Despite this, phosgene is classified as a non-persistent agent likely to be used to kill and incapacitate rather than to deny access to ground.

ABSORPTION OF PHOSGENE

Phosgene does not exert any significant effects on or via the skin. Local effects may be produced upon exposure of the eyes, and lacrimation was reported during WWI.[4] It is often assumed that phosgene is absorbed across the lung. Nash and Pattle undertook a detailed analysis of the penetration of moist biological membranes by phosgene.[6] They concluded that, given the rapidity of hydrolysis of phosgene, intact phosgene molecules would only penetrate a few tens of micrometers below such a surface. They argued that the upper respiratory tract would be significantly protected against the effects of phosgene by its surface layer of mucus but that the gas-exchange zone would be more susceptible to damage. Intact phosgene molecules might be expected to reach the pulmonary capillary blood, but once there rapid hydrolysis would occur. This is discussed in more detail below.

TOXICITY OF PHOSGENE

A great deal of work on the toxicity of phosgene in a range of species was undertaken during WWI. The toxicity of phosgene in humans is known, and a figure of 3200 mg min m^{-3} is often quoted for the LCt$_{50}$. The origin of this figure is rather obscure, and a figure of 3200 mg m^{-3} is sometimes given: this would be an LC$_{50}$ rather than an LCt$_{50}$. The variation of LCt$_{50}$ with duration of exposure has been discussed in Chapter 2; the general conformation to the Haber rule by phosgene is shown in Figure 1.

The apparent conformation to the predicted hyperbola shown in Figure 1 is, however, a little misleading: examine the data used to plot Figure 1, shown in

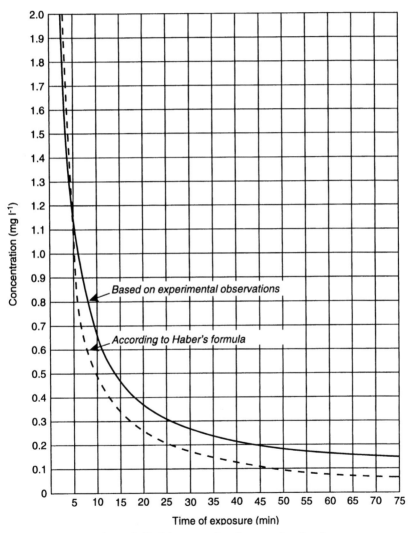

Figure 1. Toxicity curve for phosgene (on dogs)

Table 2. These data are taken from American work in dogs and mice. The lethal index shown in Table 2 is the product of concentration (expressed in mg m^{-3}) and the duration of exposure expressed in minutes. Prentiss commented that a constant lethal index would not be assumed for phosgene.[3] Data from studies undertaken during WWI are not easy to interpret: today the LCt$_{50}$ or the LC$_{50}$ would be determined (see Chapter 2); during WWI the lethal dose may have been regarded as the dose needed to ensure killing of all the animals in the study.

The toxicity of phosgene may be perhaps more usefully illustrated by the following quotation from Prentiss.[3]

a concentration of 0.50 mg per litre being fatal after 10 minutes' exposure. In higher concentrations, which are often met in battle, one or two breaths may be fatal in a few hours.

Vedder[7] may also be quoted:

as little as 1 mg per litre may be lethal if exposure lasts more than a few minutes....

Table 2. Lethal concentrations of gases (10 minutes' exposure)

Agent	American data		German data
	mg l^{-1}	Lethal index	Lethal index
Phosgene	0.50	5 000	450
Diphosgene	0.50	5 000	500
Lewisite	0.12	1 200	1 500
Mustard gas	0.15	1 500	1 500
Chloropicrin	2.00	20 000	2 000
Ethylsulphuryl chloride	1.00	10 000	2 000
Ethyldichlorarsine	0.50	5 000	3 000
Ethylbromacetate	2.30	23 000	3 000
Phenylcarbylamine chloride	0.50	5 000	3 000
Chloracetone	2.30	23 000	3 000
Benzyl iodide	3.00	30 000	3 000
Methyldichlorarsine	0.75	7 500	3 000
Acrolein	0.35	3 500	3 000
Diphenylchlorarsine	1.50	15 000	4 000
Diphenylcyanarsine	1.00	10 000	4 000
Bromacetone	3.20	32 000	4 000
Chloracetophenone	0.85	8 500	4 000
Benzyl bromide	4.50	45 000	6 000
Xylyl bromide	5.60	56 000	6 000
Brombenzyl cyanide	0.35	3 500	7 500
Chlorine	5.60	56 000	7 500
Hydrocyanic acid	0.20	2 000	1 000–4 000
Carbon monoxide	5.00	50 000	70 000

Further information on the comparative toxicity of phosgene may be found in the chapter dealing with the gas in Flury and Zernik's *War Gases*.[8]

PHARMACOLOGICAL EFFECTS OF PHOSGENE

Inhalation of phosgene produces pulmonary oedema. In the years immediately following WWI, and still in some contemporary textbooks, this was assumed to be due to the liberation of hydrochloric acid in the lung and subsequent damage to the epithelial and endothelial surfaces. Potts[5] attempted to reproduce the effects of phosgene using hydrochloric acid: interestingly, a quite different toxicological picture was produced. Inhalation of hydrochloric acid led to immediate distress and rapid death; inhalation of phosgene led to few initial effects and a delayed death. These results obtained by Potts confirmed those obtained by Winternitz in 1920.[9] Nash and Pattle demonstrated that at a phosgene concentration of 25 ppm (110.5 mg m^{-3}) the HCl produced would easily be buffered. Using a mathematical model, they calculated that the 'maximum concentration of acid in a blood–air barrier of thickness 1 μm in contact with 25 ppm of phosgene is 7×10^{-10} M which is negligible'. At very high concentrations of phosgene the production of hydrochloric acid may play a part in its toxicity; at lower levels other explanations should be sought.

Of modern theories, that of Potts,[5] in which phosgene is described as forming diamides, and that of Diller,[10] which proposed interactions between phosgene and a wide range of molecules, have proved the most persuasive. Reactions proposed by Potts and Diller are shown in Figures 2 and 3.[5]

Frosolono and Pawlowski studied biochemical changes in various lung fractions prepared from rats exposed to phosgene at concentrations near to or above the LCt$_{50}$.[11] A number of enzymes showed decreased activity in all lung fractions: these included *p*-nitrophenyl phosphatase, cytochrome *c* oxidase, ATPase and lactate dehydrogenase (LDH).

The serum LDH rose. It was suggested that either inhibition of enzyme activity or loss of enzyme from cells would account for these changes. The data available did

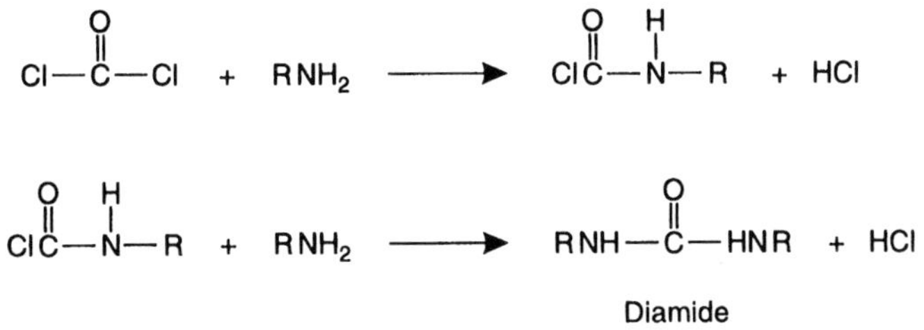

Figure 2.

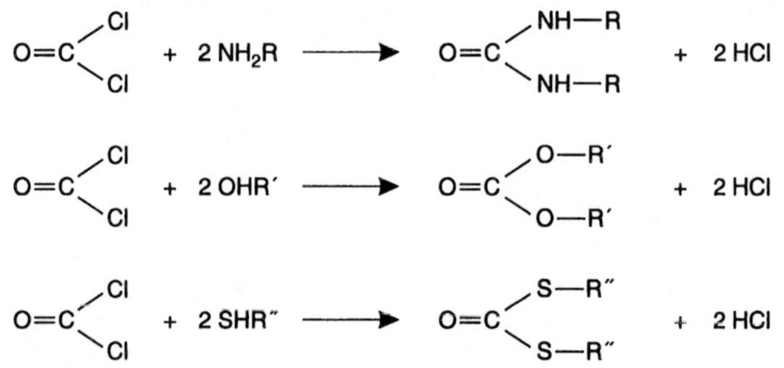

Figure 3.

not allow a distinction to be drawn between these possible mechanisms. The view that phosgene binds to essential cell components and that this leads to cell damage is now generally accepted. In 1968, however, Everett[12] revived the hydrochloric acid hypothesis and drew into the debate the earlier work of Ivanhoe.[13] It was suggested that the production of hydrochloric acid in the airways led to severe reflex bronchoconstriction and that local irritation led to pulmonary oedema. This hypothesis does not appear to have attracted general support, though the suggestion that precapillary vasoconstriction might lead to oedema has found a parallel in work on pulmonary oedema following head injury.

Exposure to very high levels of phosgene may lead to death before pulmonary oedema has developed. The cause of this is obscure, though the effect has been recorded in cases of exposure to high levels of other lung-damaging compounds, including chlorine. The hypothesis of reflex inhibition of respiration is often put forward in explanation of this effect.

THE PATHOPHYSIOLOGY OF PHOSGENE-INDUCED PULMONARY OEDEMA

The inhalation of phosgene in toxic quantities produces pulmonary oedema. The exact mechanisms involved remain remarkably obscure: in particular, the latent period (see below) is puzzling. No discussion of the effects of phosgene can be undertaken without a careful examination of current concepts of tissue fluid balance. These have changed substantially since WWI, though the early work of Starling has largely stood the test of time.[14]

It is well known that fluid tends to leak from the arterial end and to be reabsorbed at the venous end of capillaries.[15] Fluid not absorbed at the venous end of the capillaries is drained from the tissue spaces by the lymphatic system and returned to the vascular system via the lymphatic trunks which join the venous system at the root of the neck. Oedema is the accumulation of excess fluid in the tissues and may be produced by a number of causes. These include:

- an increase in hydrostatic pressure in the vascular system due perhaps to arterial hypertension or venous obstruction
- a reduction in the colloid osmotic pressure of the blood, for example in liver failure or malnutrition
- an increase in the permeability of the capillary wall as, for example, occurs in the skin as a result of the local production of, or introduction of, substances such as histamine and 5-hydroxytryptamine
- a failure of the lymphatic drainage

The balance of pressures, or forces, at the capillary wall was first described by Starling in 1896: the forces involved in controlling the movement of water across capillary walls are often referred to as the Starling forces.[14] At most capillary walls, the major ions in the plasma move freely and thus do not exert an osmotic pressure. Capillary walls are, however, much less permeable to proteins, the concentration inside capillaries being greater than the concentration in the tissue fluid. An osmotic pressure differential is, therefore, established across the capillary wall. In addition, the unequal distribution of protein anions across the capillary wall causes a Gibbs–Donnan equilibrium of ions which pass readily across the wall to be established. The combination of the osmotic pressure exerted by the protein molecules (the colloid osmotic pressure) and that contributed by the concentration difference of freely permeable ions occurring as a result of the Gibbs–Donnan equilibrium is described as the oncotic pressure of the blood.

The balance of forces across the capillary wall is expressed succinctly by the Starling equation:

$$Q_f = K_f[(P_{mv} - P_{pmv}) - \theta(\pi_{mv} - \pi_{pmv})]$$

Q_f = water flow
K_f = fluid conductance of the capillary wall
P_{mv} = intracapillary hydrostatic pressure (microvascular pressure)
P_{pmv} = tissue fluid hydrostatic pressure (perimicrovascular pressure)
π_{mv} = microvascular osmotic pressure (oncotic pressure)
π_{pmv} = perimicrovascular osmotic pressure (colloid osmotic pressure)
θ = Staverman reflection coefficient (if $\theta = 1$ then the membrane, capillary wall in this case, is completely impermeable to the molecule considered; if $\theta = 0$, then the membrane is freely permeable to the molecule considered)

In recent years understanding of the flux of water and other substances across capillary walls has been clarified by the work of A.C. Guyton and his co-workers. An excellent account of fluid balance across the pulmonary capillaries may be found in recent editions of Guyton's *Textbook of Medical Physiology*.[16] Guyton's contributions include:

- demonstration that the interstitial hydrostatic pressure is subatmospheric (sometimes referred to as 'negative')
- the concept of a safety factor which protects against the formation of oedema

The concept of the safety factor has caused some difficulty. In its simplest terms it may be thought of as the amount by which the capillary pressure has to be raised before oedema, i.e. swelling of the tissue spaces, occurs. This is a carefully constructed definition: note that it says nothing about the flow of fluid across the capillary wall—this may be substantially increased, but as long as no swelling, i.e. accumulation of water in tissue spaces, occurs, then there is no oedema.

What are the components of the safety factor? There are in fact three key components: the negative interstitial pressure, the capacity of the lymphatic system to transport more fluid than it does under normal circumstances and the fact that increased lymph drainage tends to wash protein out of the interstitial spaces, thus reducing perimicrovascular osmotic pressure.

The safety factor in the pulmonary circulation is of the order of 21 mmHg, i.e. pulmonary capillary pressure has to be raised by 21 mmHg before fluid starts to accumulate in the interstitial spaces of the lung. One cause of confusion regarding the safety factor has been the confusion alluded to above between increase of fluid flow and increase of interstitial volume. Let us examine the balance of forces across the pulmonary capillary.

Forces tending to cause movement of fluid outward from the capillaries and into the pulmonary interstitium are as follows:[16]

Capillary pressure	7 mmHg
Interstitial colloid osmotic pressure	14 mmHg
Total outward force	21 mmHg

Forces tending to cause absorption of fluid into the capillaries are as follows:[16]

Plasma colloid osmotic pressure	28 mmHg
Interstitial free fluid pressure	− 8 mmHg
Total inward force	20 mmHg
Net mean filtration pressure	+ 1 mmHg

Thus, a small net outward force exists and a constant loss of fluid from lung capillaries is to be expected. The safety factor, 21 mmHg, relates to the changes in capillary pressure which can be sustained without an increase in interstitial volume. The component of the safety factor contributed by the capacity for increased lymphatic drainage is fairly easily understood, as is the effect of washing protein out of the interstitial space. The contribution made by the negative interstitial pressure is less easy to understand. Guyton's analogy with a balloon may be helpful. Imagine a balloon connected to a vacuum pump. Let the pressure in the balloon be reduced to 10 mmHg below atmospheric. The balloon will be flat. Now turn down the vacuum pump a little until the pressure in the balloon is 5 mmHg less than atmospheric: the balloon will still be flat. Now switch off the vacuum pump and allow the balloon to equilibrate at atmospheric pressure: the balloon will still be flat. Now apply a small positive pressure (say + 1 mmHg) via the tube connected to the balloon: the balloon will expand until all the creases present when it was collapsed have disappeared. To make the balloon expand any more, positive pressure will be needed. It will be appreciated that changing the pressure inside the balloon from -10 mmHg to 0 mmHg (i.e. atmospheric pressure) produced no change in the volume of the balloon. On the contrary, changing the pressure from 0 to $+1$ mmHg produced a sudden and substantial change in volume.

Consider now the compliance of the system, recalling that compliance is defined as change in volume for unit change in pressure (dV/dP). In the negative pressure part of the curve the system has an effectively zero compliance, i.e. the balloon can withstand a change of pressure of 10 mmHg without any change in volume. However, once the internal pressure becomes positive the system displays a huge compliance: a very substantial change in volume is produced by an increase in pressure of 1 mmHg.

Guyton has demonstrated, using an isolated limb preparation in which the blood vessels were perfused with fluid of known osmotic pressure and at a given hydrostatic pressure, that a curve as shown in Figure 4 could be recorded.

We have moved some way from the pathophysiology of phosgene poisoning; let us now consider the movement of fluid across the alveolar epithelium. Guyton has suggested that the capacity of the alveolar epithelium to resist fluid flow (i.e. from the interstitial space to the intra-alveolar space) is low; indeed, he has suggested that as soon as the interstitial pressure becomes positive and the volume of the space suddenly expands (see above), fluid will flow into the alveoli. It will be understood that the negative interstitial pressure applies a draining force to the alveoli under normal conditions and the only movement of fluid into the alveoli from the interstitial space occurs as a result of capillary creep at intercellular junctions.

Fluid in the alveoli, albeit only a thin layer, will exert a force on the interstitial space. This force may be calculated by use of the law of Laplace. The law is expressed for a single spherical curved surface by the equation:

$$P + 2T/R$$

where P is the pressure exerted, T is the surface tension and R is the radius of curvature of the surface.

In the lung the radius of curvature of the alveolus is not constant: it is greater in the corners of alveoli than along the flatter parts of their walls. Also, the surface tension is not constant but varies, as a result of the special properties of surfactant, with the radius of curvature of the surface. It may be imagined that flow of fluid into the alveoli will lead to a filling of the markedly curved corners, and as the local radius of curvature is increased, a reduction in the force exerted by the lining fluid will tend to draw in more fluid. Of course, once the lining of the alveolus has formed a sphere, any further influx of fluid will reduce the radius of curvature of the surface

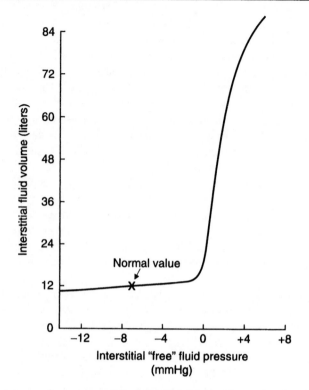

Figure 4. Pressure–volume curve of the interstitial spaces. (Extrapolated to the human being from data obtained in dogs)

and thus increase the pressure generated by the surface tension. The dilution of surfactant will raise the surface tension and thus more pressure will be generated. These mechanisms contribute to the sudden flooding of alveoli which occurs during the development of pulmonary oedema.[15]

Though some readers may think the foregoing account of pulmonary oedema is excessive, it should be recalled that it is in fact a much simplified and abbreviated account. For an excellent and detailed account the reader should consult Prichard's book *Edema of the Lung*.[17] Prichard and Lee have also contributed a valuable brief account of the topic in the *Oxford Textbook of Medicine*.[18] This account stresses the importance of pulsatile flow in the pulmonary capillaries. Movement of fluid into the interstitial space is expected during systole, but during diastole movement back into the capillaries occurs. During exercise, when the heart rate is increased, the diastole is shortened, allowing less time for return of fluid from the interstitium. Interstitial fluid pressure rises and juxtacapillary receptors are stimulated, producing the sensation of breathlessness (see below). The concept of increased efflux of fluid during exercise is of great importance in phosgene poisoning (see below).

Phosgene damages the cells of the alveolar walls and thus the alveolar–interstitial fluid barrier. Damage to the pulmonary capillaries also occurs, and the sequence of development of oedema described below supports this. Cameron and Courtice reported a series of studies on the effects of phosgene undertaken at the Chemical Defence Establishment at Porton Down (UK) during WWII.[23] Rabbits, goats and dogs were exposed to phosgene; lymph flow from the lung was measured, as was the composition of the lymph. The concentration of oedema fluid was also monitored. It was found that dogs and goats showed a marked haemoconcentration during the development of pulmonary oedema: plasma volume fell. Rabbits, however, showed little haemoconcentration despite florid pulmonary oedema. Cameron commented:

> The compensatory mechanism for rapidly restoring the plasma volume in rabbits appears to be detrimental to the life of the animal, for the more rapidly the plasma volume is restored, the more rapidly the oedema progresses. By partially dehydrating rabbits beforehand, the mortality can be decreased and haemoconcentration occurs. These observations would indicate that, in cases of haemoconcentration and fall in plasma volume due to a loss of fluid into the lungs, it would be better not to try to increase the plasma volume by transfusions, for anoxia due to pulmonary oedema is a more important factor in causing death than haemoconcentration and decreased plasma volume.

These important conclusions have been quoted at some length, as they remain of fundamental importance in the management of phosgene poisoning (see below). Whitteridge studied the effects of phosgene using an anaesthetized cat preparation.[24] A marked increase in respiratory rate and phrenic nerve activity was noted post-exposure. Later studies by Anand and Paintal confirmed that stimulation of J receptors occurred after exposure to phosgene.[25,26] Recent studies by Keeler et al. of the pathophysiology of phosgene poisoning in sheep have confirmed and extended the results of Cameron and Courtice referred to above.[27] A range of other studies of the pathophysiological effects of phosgene have been reported in recent years. Jaskot et al. have demonstrated an increase in angiotensin-converting enzyme (ACE) activity in lung tissue obtained from rats exposed to 0.5 ppm phosgene for 4 h.[28] Studies by Currie et al. have demonstrated a reduction in levels of ATP and NaK-ATPase activity in the lungs of rats also exposed to low concentrations of phosgene.[29]

Pathology of phosgene-induced lung damage

The light microscopic changes following the inhalation of phosgene were extensively studied during and after WWI. An excellent description has been provided by Winternitz.[9] The work of Meek and Eyester[19] should also be consulted, as it contains details of observations of the histopathological effects of phosgene on the dog lung made by the celebrated pulmonary anatomist William Snow Miller. Winternitz's observations have been confirmed and extended by the work of Pawlowski.[20] The chronological pattern of changes seen at the electron microscopic level may be summarized as follows:

1. The epithelium of the terminal bronchiole is the first area to be damaged. Intracellular vesiculation of both ciliated and Clara cells has been noted. This appears to be a relatively immediate effect.
2. Oedema of the alveolar interstitium appears.
3. Intracellular oedema of the cells of the interalveolar septa appears.
4. Focal disruption of alveolar type I cells noted.
5. Marked swelling of interalveolar septa observed.
6. Appearance of frank intra-alveolar oedema.

The oedema fluid is eosinophilic at light microscopy and contains much protein. It seems unlikely that phosgene attacks one particular cell type in the lung. The resistance of the thin part of the blood–air barrier to attack by phosgene has been noted but no deductions regarding protective mechanisms or mechanisms of damage seem to have been drawn.

The pattern described above is the common one seen in many types of permeability pulmonary oedema. This has been described and discussed in detail by Staub, Teplitz and Robin.[15,21,22] The account provided by Prichard is of great value.[18]

SYMPTOMS AND SIGNS OF PHOSGENE POISONING

Extensive descriptions of the symptoms and signs of phosgene poisoning may be found in the accounts of Ireland,[4] Vedder,[7] Diller,[10] Everett,[12] Seidelin,[30] Fruhmann[31] and Cucinell.[32]

During or immediately after exposure to dangerous concentrations of phosgene the following symptoms and signs develop: eye irritation, respiratory tract irritation, lacrimation, coughing, a feeling of choking and tightness in the chest. In some cases nausea, retching and vomiting have been reported. The severity of these early effects is, however, no guide to the severity of the poisoning: patients who may later die may show minimal or no symptoms or signs at the time of exposure. An effect frequently reported during WWI was the 'tobacco reaction': men who had inhaled only a small quantity of phosgene reported a flat metallic taste upon lighting a cigarette. This reaction has also been reported in cases of hydrogen cyanide and sulphur dioxide poisoning but is ill-understood.

Following exposure to phosgene, a latent period ranging from 30 min to 24 h may occur before the onset of more serious symptoms and signs. The onset of these may be precipitated by exercise, and collapse of patients exposed to phosgene on subsequently taking exercise was frequently reported during WWI.[4] Once the latent period is over, patients develop dyspnoea, a painful cough and cyanosis. Increasing quantities of frothy white or yellowish fluid may be expectorated. Later the fluid tends to become pink-tinged. A mushroom-like efflux of pink foam ('Champignon d'écume': mushroom of foam or froth) may appear at the mouth in the dying. On physical examination diminished breath sounds and rales and ronche in all areas may be detected. The blood pressure may be low and the heart rate raised to more than 130 per minute. Circulatory collapse and cardiac failure may occur.

Of fatal cases 80% may be expected to die during the first 24–48 h post-exposure. Deaths during WWI in patients who had survived this initial period were often as a result of pneumonia. Selgrade *et al.* have shown that exposure to low concentrations of phosgene (0.25 ppm for 4 h) significantly increased mortality rates on post-exposure challenge with aerosolized *Streptococcus zooepidimicus.*[33] An account of a case of phosgene poisoning is reproduced below.[34]

February 3 1917: A chemist was working at a new chemical product. A syphon of phosgene, required for the synthesis of this substance, burst on his table at 1.00 pm. A yellowish cloud was seen by a second person in the room to go up close to the chemist's face, who exclaimed, 'I am gassed' and both hurried out of the room. Outside, the patient sat down on a chair looking pale and coughing slightly.

2.30 pm: In bed at hospital, to which he had been taken by car, having been kept at rest since the accident. Hardly coughing at all, pulse normal. No distress or anxiety and talking freely to friends for over an hour. During this time he was so well that the medical officer was not even asked to see the patient upon admission to hospital.

5.30 pm: Coughing with frothy expectoration commenced and the patient was noticed to be bluish about the lips. His condition now rapidly deteriorated. Every fit of coughing brought up large quantities of clear, yellowish frothy fluid of which about 80 ounces were expectorated in one and a half hours. His face became a grey ashen colour, never purple, though the pulse remained fairly strong. He died at 6.50 pm without any great struggle for breath. The symptoms of irritation were very slight at the onset; there was then a delay of at least four hours and the final development of serious oedema up to death took little more than an hour though the patient was continually rested in bed.

MANAGEMENT OF PHOSGENE POISONING

A number of deductions regarding the proper management of phosgene poisoning may be drawn from the discussion of the pathophysiology of phosgene poisoning; this should be borne in mind in the following section.

As usual in cases of exposure to chemical warfare agents, management of phosgene poisoning may be divided into two parts, first aid measures and therapy.

First aid measure

The casualty should be removed from the source of the phosgene. Rescue workers should wear adequate respiratory protection. Decontamination of casualties is not necessary.

Therapy

A comprehensive account of the various approaches which have been used in the treatment of phosgene poisoning may be found in the papers presented at a recent symposium.[35] One of the standard rules laid down during WWI for the management of phosgene casualties was that the casualties should undertake no exercise and should be given complete rest as soon as possible. The effect of exercise on the efflux of fluid from pulmonary capillaries to the pulmonary interstitium has already been considered. Detailed experimental studies by Postel et al., however, indicated that at least in some species exercise did not have a marked effect on the outcome of phosgene poisoning.[36] This was particularly the case in rats and mice, though in dogs exercise after phosgene poisoning increased lung weight beyond that seen in the poisoned but rested controls. In clinical practice, bed rest is invariably recommended.

Patients presenting with cyanosis and PaO_2 levels of less than 50 mmHg require additional oxygen in their inspired air. Depending on the severity of lung damage, oxygen may be administered by face-mask or endotracheal tube. Positive end expiratory pressure may be needed to achieve adequate oxygenation. An early recommendation that inspired gases should be passed through 90% ethyl alcohol to reduce frothing of airway secretions does not seem to be followed today.

During WWI great emphasis was placed on the value of oxygen in the treatment of phosgene poisoning. The following extract is taken from *The Official History of the Great War: Medical Services; Diseases of War*, Vol II:[34]

> Oxygen should always be given to casualties with serious pulmonary oedema, that is to men with intense blue cyanosis or grey pallor. These need oxygen continuously and over a long period. If the supply permits of such use, it should be given also to milder cases of oedema in order to prevent their lapsing into a more serious state of asphyxia. It should be remembered that in every autopsy on early death from pulmonary irritant poisoning, extreme oedema of the lungs was found, that cyanosis is the main indication of such oedema, and that no case in whom it was possible to restore a pink colour by the proper use of oxygen died of this pulmonary oedema.

Such therapy was recommended by those exceptionally experienced in treating phosgene poisoning on a large scale. Further details may be found in the works of Haldane[37] and Barcroft.[38]

Rest and oxygen, then, are the mainstays of management: drugs are of secondary value.

DRUG TREATMENT

Steroids

The use of large doses of steroids has become standard in the management of permeability pulmonary oedema. There is considerable experimental evidence to suggest that steroids given to experimental animals before exposure to pulmonary-oedema-inducing agents can ameliorate the oedema. This presumably is linked with the inhibition of the inflammatory response to the irritant. Evidence for the value of steroids after exposure to phosgene and other lung-damaging compounds is weak. However, if steroids are to be given they should be given:

- as soon as possible after exposure
- in large doses
- discontinued fairly quickly

Methylprednisolone sodium succinate has been proposed, in the following regime:

- 15 min or less post-exposure: 2000 mg IV or IM
- 6 h post-exposure: 2000 mg IV or IM
- 12 h post-exposure: 2000 mg IV or IM

Continue at the same dose 12 hourly for 1–5 days, depending on the patient's condition.[2]

A number of reports of the value of steroids and some suggesting that they are of little value are noted below.

Everett reported the successful use of hydrocortisone (200 mg per day) in a case of phosgene poisoning.[12] Diller considered that the use of steroids was indicated in phosgene poisoning and suggested that inhibition of prostaglandin generation and release, inhibition of leukocyte release of kinins, inhibition of proteolysis and stabilization of mucopolysaccharides leading to maintenance of normal capillary permeability might underlie their effectiveness.[10] Bradley, on the other hand, felt that their evidence for the efficacy of steroids in phosgene poisoning was inconclusive, though he used methylprednisolone in the case reported in his paper.[39] The administration of steroids by inhalation has also been recommended.[2]

In 1987, Prichard and Lee summed up current opinion on the value of steroids in the management of permeability pulmonary oedema in their valuable chapter in the *Oxford Textbook of Medicine*.[18] Their final paragraph on the point concluded:

> [regarding the use of steroids in high-permeability pulmonary oedema] However, there is some logic in their use, for evidence is now very strong that granulocytes aggregate in the lungs of patients with ARDS as a result of complement activation. Steroids can not only reduce their aggregation but also diminish free radical production. Until a conclusive answer is produced, clinicians will continue to use steroids in large doses despite the absence of adequate supportive clinical data.

The need for a clinical trial of the value of steroids in the management of phosgene poisoning is clear.

Antibiotics

The use of prophylactic antibiotics in cases of phosgene poisoning has often been recommended: penicillin G, amoxycillin and chloramphenicol have all been used.[10,12]

Other drugs which have been recommended

- Aminophylline[12]
- Dopamine[39]
- Codeine phosphate for alleviation of cough[2]
- ε-Aminocaproic acid[10]
- Phosgene antiserum[40]

Hexamethylenetetramine (HMT or methenamine or hexamine or urotropine)

The history of the use of HMT to alleviate or prevent the effects of phosgene is a long one. In designing respirators to defend against phosgene during WWI a range of compounds was examined. Soda lime (a mixture of sodium hydroxide and calcium hydroxide) proved effective. Phenol and sodium phenolate were also effective, and British Phenolate Helmet (P Helmet) was first used on 15 December 1915. This was followed by the Phenolate Hexamine Helmet (P.H. Helmet) from early 1916 onwards. The P.H. Helmets comprised a flannel sack which had been dipped in a mixture of sodium phenolate and hexamine. The discovery that hexamine neutralized phosgene was made in Russia.[3] The addition of goggles to the P.H. Helmet provided considerable protection against lacrimatory agents as well as against phosgene; such helmets lasted for about 24 h of continuous use.

These chemically reactive masks were replaced by canister respirators fairly quickly: canisters containing lime and charcoal proved very effective in removing a wide range of chemical agents from the inspired air. Those interested in the development of respirators should consult Prentiss's excellent account.[3]

Hexamine still figures in the British National Formulary (as methenamine hippurate) as a long-term treatment for urinary tract infections.[41] Hexamine was long considered as likely to be of little value in the management of phosgene poisoning: rather as in the case of steroids, it was accepted that there was a case for its likely efficacy if given to experimental animals prior to exposure to phosgene but that it would not be likely to be effective when given after exposure had occurred. In 1971, Stravrakis challenged this view and reported several cases where hexamine had been given (20 ml of a 20% solution IV) as soon as possible after exposure to phosgene.[42] The author felt that the treatment had been of value and stated:

> If given intravenously during the latent period soon after exposure, hexamethylene-tetramine will adequately protect the victim of phosgene exposure.

Diller held, on the contrary, that there was no evidence in the form of adequately controlled experiments to support the assertion that hexamine is of value when administered after phosgene exposure.[10,43] Diller's 1980 account is a valuable source of references to earlier papers on hexamine.[43]

Few clinicians today would recommend the use of hexamine in the management of phosgene poisoning.

LONG-TERM EFFECTS OF EXPOSURE TO PHOSGENE

Chronic bronchitis and emphysema have been reported as consequences of phosgene exposure.[32] Diller suggested that the great majority of patients who recovered after an exposure to phosgene would make a complete recovery.[44] He noted that exertional dyspnoea had been reported and this sometimes took some time (months) to resolve. This has also been reported after exposure to mustard gas.

REFERENCES

1. Lefebure V (1921) *The Riddle of the Rhine*. London: W. Collins Sons & Co., Ltd.
2. Ministry of Defence (1987) *Medical Manual of Defence Against Chemical Agents*. Ministry of Defence D/Med(F & S) (2)/10/1/1. London: HMSO.
3. Prentiss AM (1937) *Chemicals in War*. New York: McGraw-Hill Book Company Inc.
4. Ireland MM (1926) *Medical Aspects of Gas Warfare*. Vol. XIV of the *Medical Department of the United States on the World War*. Washington DC: US Government.
5. Potts AM, Simon FP and Gerard RW (1949) The mechanism of action of phosgene and diphosgene. *Arch Biochem*, **24**, 329–337.
6. Nash T and Pattle RE (1971) The absorption of phosgene by aqueous solutions and its relation to toxicity. *Ann Occup Hyg*, **51**, 303–320.
7. Vedder EB (1925) *The Medical Aspects of Chemical Warfare*. Baltimore: Williams & Wilkins Co.
8. Flury F and Zernik F (1931) Phosgen. In: *Schüdische Gase*, pp. 222–228. Berlin.
9. Winternitz MC (1920) *Pathology of War Gas Poisoning*. New Haven: Yale University Press.
10. Diller WF (1978) Medical phosgene problems and their possible solution. *J Occup Med*, **20**, 189–193.
11. Frosolono MF and Pawlowski R (1977) Effect of phosgene on rat lungs after single high-level exposure. I. Biochemical alterations. *Arch Environ Health*, **32**, 271–277.
12. Everett ED and Overholt EL (1968) Phosgene poisoning. *JAMA*, **205**, 243–245.
13. Ivanhoe F and Meyers FH (1964) Phosgene poisoning as an example of neuroparalytic acute pulmonary edema: the sympathetic vasomotor reflex involved. *Dis Chest*, **46**, 211–218.
14. Starling EH (1896) On the absorption of fluid from connective tissue spaces. *J Physiol*, **19**, 312–336.
15. Staub NC (1974) Pulmonary oedema. *Physiol Rev*, **54**, 678–811.
16. Guyton AC (1986) *Textbook of Medical Physiology*, 7th edn. Philadelphia, London: WB Saunders.
17. Prichard JS (1982) *Edema of the Lung*. Springfield, Illinois: Charles C. Thomas.
18. Prichard JS and Lee G de J (1987) Pulmonary oedema. In: *Oxford Textbook of Medicine* (DJ Weatherall, JGG Ledingham and DA Worrell, eds), Chapter 13. Oxford: Oxford University Press.
19. Meek WJ and Eyster JAE (1920) Experiments on the pathological physiology of acute phosgene poisoning. *Am J Physiol*, **51**, 303–320.
20. Pawlowski R and Frosolono MF (1977) Effect of phosgene on rat lungs after single high-level exposure. II. Ultrastructural alterations. *Arch Environ Health*, **32**, 278–283.
21. Teplitz C (1979) Pulmonary cellular and interstitial oedema. In: *Pulmonary Oedema* (AP Fishman and EM Renkin, eds), pp. 97–112. Bethesda, Maryland: American Physiology Society.

22. Robin ED (1979) Permeability pulmonary oedema. In: *Pulmonary Oedema* (AP Fishman and EM Renkin, eds), pp. 217–228. Bethesda, Maryland: American Physiological Society.

23. Cameron GR and Courtice FC (1946) The production and removal of oedema fluid in the lung after exposure to carbonyl chloride (phosgene). *J Physiol*, **105**, 175–185.

24. Whitteridge D (1948) The action of phosgene on the stretch receptors of the lung. *J Physiol*, **107**, 107–114.

25. Anand A, Paintal AS and Whitteridge D (1986) Phosgene stimulates J receptors and produces increased respiratory drive in cats. *J Physiol*, **371**, 1098.

26. Paintal AS (1969) Mechanisms of stimulation of type J pulmonary receptors. *J Physiol*, **203**, 511–532.

27. Keeler JR, Hurt HH, Nold JB *et al.* (1990) Phosgene-induced lung injury in sheep. *Inhalation Toxicol*, **2**, 391–406.

28. Jaskot RH, Grose EC and Stead AG (1989) Increase in angiotensin-converting enzyme in rat lungs following inhalation of phosgene. *Inhalation Toxicol*, **1**, 71–78.

29. Currie WD, Pratt PC and Frosolono MF (1985) Response of pulmonary energy metabolism to phosgene. *Toxicol Ind Health*, **1**, 17–27.

30. Seidelin R (1961) The inhalation of phosgene in a fire extinguisher accident. *Thorax*, **16**, 91–93.

31. Fruhmann G (1974) Die Behandlung des Lungenödems nach Reizgasinhalation. (Treatment of pulmonary edema following inhalation of irritant gas.) *Ther Gegegnw*, **113**, 38–46.

32. Cucinell SA (1974) Review of the toxicity of long-term phosgene exposure. *Arch Environ Health*, **28**, 272–275.

33. Selgrade MK, Starnes DM, Illing JW *et al.* (1989) Effects of phosgene exposure on bacterial, viral and neoplastic lung disease susceptibility in mice. *Inhalation Toxicol*, **1**, 243–259.

34. Vedder EB (1923) In: *History of The Great War. Medical Services. Diseases of the War.* Vol. II (WG MacPherson, WP Herringham, TR Elliott and A Balfour, eds), p. 390. London: HMSO.

35. Mehlman MA, Fensterheim RJ and Frosolono MF (1985) Phosgene induced edema: diagnosis and therapeutic countermeasures. An international symposium. *Toxicol Ind Health*, **1**, 1–160.

36. Postel S, Tobias JM, Patt HM *et al.* (1946) The effect of exercise on mortality of animals poisoned with diphosgene. *Proc Soc Exp Biol Med*, **63**, 432–436.

37. Haldane JS (1919) Lung-irritant gas poisoning and its sequelae. *J R Army Med Coll*, **33**, 494–507.

38. Barcroft J (1920) Discussion on the therapeutic uses of oxygen. *Proc R Soc Med London*, **XIII**, 59–99.

39. Bradley BL and Unger KM (1982) Phosgene inhalation: a case report. *Texas Med*, **78**, 51–53.

40. Ong SG (1972) Treatment of phosgene poisoning with antiserum anaphylactic shock by phosgene. *Arch Toxicol*, **29**, 267–278.

41. Joint Formulary Committee. British Medical Association. Pharmaceutical Society of Great Britain (1993) *British National Formulary*: BNF Number 25. London: British Medical Association.

42. Stavrakis P (1971) The use of hexamethylenetetramine (HMT) in treatment of phosgene poisoning. *Ind Med*, **40**, 30–31.

43. Diller WF (1980) The methenamine misunderstanding in the therapy of phosgene poisoning. *Arch Toxicol*, **46**, 199–206.

44. Diller WF (1985) Late sequelae after phosgene poisoning: a literature review. *Toxicol Ind Health*, **1**, 129–133.

9

CYANIDES

Three chemical warfare (CW) compounds are important under this heading: (1) hydrogen cyanide (HCN), (2) cyanogen chloride and (3) cyanogen bromide. They are sometimes known as 'blood agents', although the blood is not a main site of their toxic effects. All three share their main toxic properties, but cyanogen chloride and bromide are additionally irritant to the respiratory tract. HCN has not been particularly successful as a CW agent, and the high volatility of the compound precluded its use on a large scale in World War I. Attempts were made to produce more effective munitions by making mixtures: one such was Vincennite, which contained 50% HCN, 30% arsenic trichloride, 15% stannic chloride and 5% chloroform. Modern chemical weapons might enable an intensive strike using HCN-laden munitions, in which case HCN could be used more successfully. As with many other chemical weapons, successful use of HCN would depend upon the element of surprise. Well-protected troops would withstand such an attack well: unprotected troops or civilians would not.

Because HCN disperses rapidly, it is classed as a non-persistent agent.

HCN was used for mass extermination in Germany during World War II. The material used by the German authorities was Zyklon B, made by IG Farben. Zyklon B briquettes were calcium sulfate impregnated with HCN and were 40% HCN by weight. Cyanide has also been used for assassination.

PHYSICAL PROPERTIES

The physical properties of HCN are shown in Table 1. Below 26°C, HCN is a colorless or yellow-brown liquid. It is unstable as usually prepared but the highly purified material is reputed to be stable. On standing it polymerizes and may explode. It can be stabilized with phosphoric acid.

HCN is variously described as smelling of bitter almonds, marzipan, ratafia or peach kernels. While some can smell HCN at very low concentrations,[1] others cannot smell HCN at all.

Table 1. Physical properties of HCN

Molecular weight	27.02
Boiling point	26°C
Melting point	−14°C
Vapor density	0.93 compared to air
Density of liquid	0.697 at 10°C
Vapor pressure	165 mmHg at −10°C
	256 mmHg at 0°C
	600 mmHg at 20°C
	757 mmHg at 26°C

ROUTE OF EXPOSURE

Under CW conditions, HCN is likely to exist in the form of a gas. Thus the route of exposure would be by inhalation. It should be noted that liquid HCN is rapidly absorbed across the skin.

MODE OF ACTION

The main toxic action is due to the inhibition of cytochrome oxidase,[2] interfering with aerobic respiration at the cellular level.[3] The cells are fully oxygenated but cannot utilize the oxygen. The result is the accumulation of lactic acid, and cell death occurs from histotoxic anoxia. The role of calcium influx in cyanide-induced neuronal cell death has been investigated.[4,5]

TOXICOLOGY

Acute toxicity

Precise figures for the acute toxicity of HCN to humans are unknown. The acute lethality is, by analogy with animals and on theoretical grounds, likely to be time dependent and some guideline figures are available in Table 2. However, it should be

Table 2. Inhalation toxicity to humans: guideline figures

Time	LC_{50} (mg m^{-3})	LCt_{50} (mg min m^{-3})
15 s	2400	660
1 min	1000	1000
10 min	200	2000
15 min	133	4000

stated that these figures are extremely uncertain, and a higher figure of 4400 mg m^{-3} for the LC$_{50}$ was given by MacNamara,[6] based on an estimate of Moore and Gates, who used the following formula to relate intravenous LD$_{50}$ to LCt$_{50}$:

$$VaC - Dt = K$$

where

V = volume of HCN inhaled (l kg^{-1})
a = fraction absorbed
C = concentration of HCN (mg^{-1})
D = rate of detoxication (0.17 mg kg^{-1} min^{-1})
K = LD$_{50}$ for injected cyanide

MacNamara's own estimates for the toxicity of inhaled HCN in humans is based on the similarity in responses to HCN of humans and goats, and he gives a 1-min LC$_{50}$ of 3404 mg m^{-3}.

Comparative aspects

There are considerable interspecies differences in acute single-dose toxicity of HCN. The reasons for this are complex but include differences in metabolic rate, in detoxication rate and in the degree of respiratory stimulation produced by HCN: for discussion see Barcroft[7] and MacNamara.[6]

It is important to note that cyanides are subject to an endogenous detoxication system, and only when the body is presented with cyanide at a rate which overwhelms the system will poisoning occur. Detoxication is carried out by the enzymes rhodanese (thiosulfate-cyanide sulfurtransferase) and to a lesser extent β-mercaptopyruvate-cyanide sulfurtransferase. The sulfurtransferases use sulfur donors to produce thiocyanate, which is much less toxic than cyanide. There is also evidence for oxidative detoxication and combination with endogenous cobalamins.[8] The result is that the toxicity of cyanides is strongly dependent upon dose rate and therefore, in the case of inhaled cyanides, concentration. Thus HCN does not obey Haber's law ($Ct = K$). In acute cyanide poisoning it is unlikely that detoxication plays any significant role, but the existence of pathways for detoxication explains the ability of animals to withstand low concentrations of cyanide indefinitely.

Symptoms and signs

Qualitatively, the clinical signs and symptoms of HCN poisoning in humans and animals are similar. The most notable feature of HCN poisoning by inhalation is its extremely rapid onset, which is a consequence of the rapid distribution of cyanide.[9] The first sign is hyperventilation in most species, including humans,[6] and this, of course, increases the dose inhaled at any given concentration. Hyperventilation is followed by loss of consciousness and convulsions: the corneal reflex is lost and death occurs from cardiac and/or respiratory arrest.[6,8,10] HCN is rapidly absorbed and blood levels start to fall on cessation of exposure; therefore, if the dose of HCN has not produced lethal blood levels, and if further exposure is avoided, the animal will usually recover without antidotes.[8,9] Exposure to lower doses produces a less dramatic clinical picture; the odor of almonds may be noted and there is a feeling of apprehension. A metallic taste in the mouth has been remarked upon, and dyspnea occurs at quite low concentrations.

The comparative effects of HCN on humans and dogs was studied by the distinguished physiologist Joseph Barcroft.[6] Barcroft entered a chamber containing HCN accompanied by a dog. The chamber contained HCN at a concentration of between $1/2000$ and $1/1600$; $1/2000 = 500$ ppm (approximately 500 mg m^{-3}). Barcroft tried to be about as active as the dog. After about 30 s the dog became unsteady. At about 55 s, the dog fell to the floor and commenced the distressing respiration which precedes death from cyanide poisoning. About 95 s after the experiment started, the dog's body was carried out, respiration having ceased. Barcroft left the chamber, the only effect on him being momentary giddiness on turning the head. He had subsequent difficulty in concentration for about a year.

The experiment appeared conclusive, though this was marred by the finding that the dog, set aside for burial, was walking about, apparently normal, the next morning and also showed no further signs. Some doubt has been cast on the concentration of HCN to which Barcroft was exposed, in the light of his almost complete absence of symptoms.

Vedder in 1925[11] contributed a useful account of the effects of acute exposure to high concentrations of HCN:

> In an atmosphere containing a lethal concentration an odour of bitter almonds is noticed. This is followed by a sensation of constriction of the throat, giddiness confusion and indistinct sight. The head feels as though the temples were gripped in a vice, and there may be pain in the back of the neck, pain in the chest, with palpitation and laboured respiration. Unconsciousness occurs and the man drops. From this moment if the subject remains in the atmosphere of hydrocyanic acid for more than two or three minutes death almost always ensues, after a brief period of convulsions followed by failure of respiration.
>
> (Vedder EB (1925) *The Medical Aspects of Chemical Warfare*. Baltimore: William & Wilkins)

Delayed toxicity

Even where sodium or potassium salts are responsible, most cases of human cyanide poisoning are fatal. This is even more the case with HCN, which might be used in chemical warfare, and which is much more quickly absorbed by inhalation than are the salts when ingested. Both in humans and in experimental animals, survivors can suffer long-term effects, presumably where the dose is close to a lethal one. Such effects are often rather vague and include intellectual deterioration, mental confusion and parkinsonism.[12–16] Somewhat surprisingly, slow partial recovery of intellectual capacity over a period of years has been described.[12]

Pathological changes can be produced in experimental animals and observed in human cyanide poisonings which appear to be correlated with these delayed effects. Thus lesions in the white matter have been produced in rats,[17] and in gray and white matter in rats,[18] dogs[19,20] and cats.[21] However, Haymaker *et al.*[19] stated that the gray matter was more severely affected after survival of single doses and the white matter after multiple sublethal injection. Finelli's patient (see above), who ingested a cyanide-containing insecticide, was shown to have globus pallidus infarction upon computed tomography.

Chronic toxicity

The various syndromes such as tropical ataxic neuropathy[22] associated with chronic administration of low doses of cyanide have no relevance to the effects of the use of HCN in warfare.

Diagnosis of HCN poisoning postmortem

There is no gross or microscopical feature that is unique to cyanide poisoning,[23] and where death supervenes rapidly only cerebral edema is constantly reported.[24] The cherry-red appearance of the blood and organs, because of the fully oxygenated state of the body, has often been remarked upon, but this sign is inconstant and frequently not obvious. Blood and tissue cyanide concentrations are the investigations most likely to be helpful, but these are less and less helpful with the passage of time since death.[25] This is because of a combination of postmortem cyanogenesis and postmortem transulfuration. Factors such as smoking render blood and urine thiocyanate concentrations difficult to interpret.

MANAGEMENT

As HCN is very rapidly absorbed by the inhalation route and blood levels start to fall when exposure ceases, if the dose of HCN has not produced blood levels in the lethal range, and if further exposure does not take place, the casualty will usually recover without antidotes.[8,9] Even where use of antidotes is appropriate, general measures will be of great importance. Despite the often-repeated adage that oxygen is of no value in cyanide poisoning, as the body is fully oxygenated, a number of studies have shown slight but reproducible evidence that oxygen is beneficial.

First aid

The casualty should be removed from the source of HCN. This is the single most important measure. Decontamination of casualties is unlikely to be necessary because of the volatility of HCN.

Antidotes

A number of antidotes are available for cyanide (see Table 3) and there are marked differences in therapeutic attitudes in different countries (Table 4). This is sometimes said to be a reflection of the fact that no antidote is completely satisfactory, but the differing national attitudes partly reflect the influence and nationality of scientists in this area of work. Moreover, many of the antidotes are very successful in experimental studies, and the poor clinical results primarily reflect the difficulty of treating a poisoning of such rapid onset. All the antidotal regimes use either the principle of enhanced enzymic detoxication (e.g. sodium thiosulfate), direct binding of cyanide (cobalt compounds) or indirect binding (the methemoglobin generators).

SULFUR DONORS AND RHODANESE

Sodium thiosulfate

Sodium thiosulfate forms, with sodium nitrite, the 'classical therapy' for cyanide poisoning. Its action is to hasten the enzymic detoxication of cyanide by supplying a source of sulfane sulfur for the enzyme rhodanese,[38] which detoxifies cyanide to thiocyanate. The rate of activity of this enzyme is limited by availability of sulfane sulfur. Sodium thiosulfate, which is not the natural cosubstrate for the enzyme, can increase the rate of transulfuration up to 30-fold,[39,40] despite the poor access of the drug to the mitochondria and the location of rhodanese in that organelle. Nevertheless, by itself thiosulfate causes blood cyanide levels to fall only slowly and this antidote is therefore used as a second-line cyanide antidote, usually with a methemoglobin generator.

The reaction can be represented as:

$$Na_2S_2O_3 + CN^- \rightarrow SCN^- + Na_2SO_3$$

The usual dose of sodium thiosulfate is 50 ml of the 25% solution.

Other sulfur donors and rhodanese

Attempts have been made to bring about the co-location of the sulfur donor and the enzyme in the same fluid compartment. Two approaches have been adopted: (1) parenteral injection of the enzyme so that it is present in the extracellular fluid; (2) use of sulfur donors more capable of crossing membranes. Injected rhodanese, usually of beef liver origin,[41,42] has been used in experimental studies. In these studies it was found that the small antidotal effect of thiosulfate was considerably improved by rhodanese. Alternative sulfur donors have included the sodium salts of ethanethiosulfonic acid and propanethiosulfonic acid. By comparison with sodium thiosulfate any superiority observed has been small, but combined with rhodanese a greater advantage was seen.[42] However, none of these alternative sulfur donors has reached clinical practice. A further approach along these lines has been the use of rhodanese and sodium thiosulfate, microencapsulated in mouse erythrocytes.[43]

Table 3. Approaches to the antidotal therapy of HCN poisoning: antidotes in clinical use are in italics

Hastening the enzymic detoxication of cyanide
  Sulfur donors
    Sodium thiosulfate
    Sodium ethanethiosulfonate
    Sodium propanethiosulfonate
    Sodium mercaptopyruvate[26]
    Sodium tetrathionate[27]
  Exogenous sulfurtransferases
    Rhodanese
      Bovine heart
      Bacterial
    β-mercaptopyruvate cyanide sulfurtransferase
Complexation with heavy metals
  Cobalt
    Dicobalt edetate
    Cobaltous chloride
    Cobaltous acetate
    Cobalt histidine
    Sodium cobaltinitrite*[28,29]
    Hydroxocobalamin
  Iron
    Endogenous methemoglobin generated by
      Sodium nitrite
      Amyl nitrite
      4-Dimethylaminophenol
      Compounds primarily of interest in prophylaxis
        4-Aminopropiophenone
        (*p*-aminopropiophenone, PAPP)
        Hydroxylamine[30]
    Exogenous methemoglobin
Carbohydrates and related compounds
  Glucose
  Sodium pyruvate
  α-Oxoglutaric acid[31]
  Glyceraldehyde
  Pyridoxal 5-phosphate[32]
Drugs that do not directly interact with cyanide
  Chlorpromazine[33]
  Etomidate
  Naloxone[34]
  Meclofenoxate (centrophenoxone)[35]
  Phenoxybenzamine[36,37]

*Also a methemoglobin generator.

Table 4. Antidotal regimes for cyanide poisoning

Country	Regime
USA	Sodium nitrite + sodium thiosulfate
UK*, France†	Dicobalt edetate
Germany	4-Dimethylaminophenol + sodium thiosulfate

*Cyanide antidote kits available in the UK generally contain sodium nitrite and thiosulfate in addition to dicobalt edetate.
†Much of the impetus towards the use of hydroxocobalamin has come from France.

Another enzymic pathway known to play a part in the detoxification of cyanide has been exploited experimentally, namely the β-mercaptopyruvate:cyanide sulfurtransferase route of detoxification. In these studies, sodium β-mercaptopyruvate was investigated as an antidote.

COMPLEXATION WITH HEAVY METALS

Cyanide forms stable complexes of low toxicity with many heavy metal ions, notably iron and cobalt, but also silver, chromium and rhodium.[44] The usual source of iron in the treatment of cyanide poisoning is methemoglobin generated by chemical means from the patient's own hemoglobin, using compounds such as the nitrites or 4-dimethylaminophenol. In contrast, cobalt is usually used in the form of injectable dicobalt edetate.

TREATMENT OF HCN POISONING BY METHEMOGLOBIN FORMATION

Methemoglobinemia is a generally undesirable condition, in which the Fe^{2+} in erythrocytic hemoglobin is oxidized to Fe^{3+}. High levels of methemeglobin are life-threatening, as hemoglobin in the oxidized form is unable to carry oxygen. However, methemoglobin has the property of combining with certain noxious anions, including cyanide, rendering them less toxic, and therapeutic methemoglobinemias in the region of 30–40% seem to be fairly safe. The cyanide is effectively sequestrated inside the red cell as a complex, namely cyanmethemoglobin. In the treatment of cyanide poisoning, the usual way of generating the methemoglobinemia is the use of chemicals, although injectable exogenous stroma-free methemoglobin has been studied in experimental animals.[45,46]

Methemoglobin is reduced to hemoglobin by erythrocytic methemoglobin reductase so that chemical methemoglobinemia is a temporary phenomenon. The reduction of methemoglobin to hemoglobin causes the binding of cyanide to be of limited duration. This would mean that cyanide would eventually start diffusing out of the red cell. As the endogenous detoxication of cyanide cannot be relied upon to produce adequate detoxication of cyanide before the methemoglobinemia is reversed, a second antidote is necessary, almost always sodium thiosulfate. To use chemically generated methemoglobinemia safely to treat cyanide poisoning, it is important to note that commonly used methods for measuring that pigment measure cyanmethemoglobin as ordinary hemoglobin, which will give a falsely optimistic level for the remaining fraction of blood pigment which can reversibly carry oxygen. Furthermore, there are individuals with rare inherited methemoglobinemias: these may be at risk of developing abnormally high levels of methemoglobin in response to therapeutic methemoglobin generators.

Nitrites

The efficacy of amyl nitrite in cyanide poisoning was first noted in 1888 by Pedigo.[47] In experimental animals, inhalation of amyl nitrate can give rise to substantial levels of methemoglobin[48] and successfully antagonize several multiples of a lethal dose of cyanide.[49] In contrast, only low levels of methemoglobin seem generally to be produced in humans,[50] although some case reports suggest otherwise.[51] The probable reason for this is that it is not possible to persuade human volunteers to inhale doses comparable to those that can be administered to experimental animals. Despite doubts over its efficacy, amyl nitrite ampoules (0.2 or 0.3 ml) are frequently used in acute cyanide poisoning. Sodium nitrite was introduced in the 1920s and the combination of sodium nitrite and thiosulfate in the 1930s.[52]

This combination is often referred to as the 'classical therapy' for cyanide poisoning. A notable feature, in experimental studies, is the marked synergism between the two components of the classical therapy,[53] and a combination of sodium nitrite and thiosulfate remains the standard treatment in many countries, including the USA, the usual adult dose of sodium nitrite being 300 mg in 10 ml given intravenously. The classical therapy has been superseded by dicobalt edetate in the UK and France on the basis of animal studies that showed the cobalt compound to be more effective or to have a better therapeutic index.[54,55] Sodium nitrite has been superseded in Germany by 4-dimethylaminophenol (DMAP) on the basis that the latter compound generates methemoglobin more quickly. However, it should be noted that it has been claimed that sodium nitrite does not exert its action entirely through the generation of methemoglobin.[56]

Sodium nitrite, like all methemoglobin producers, is apt to cause hypoxia in overdose, and repeated administration reduces red cell survival. Furthermore, sodium nitrite causes vasodilatation and a drop in the blood pressure. However, many of the reports that led to sodium nitrite being superseded are irrelevant to the use of sodium nitrite in a CW scenario. This is because they relate to children[57,58] or newborn animals.[59]

Aminophenols

It has been known for many years that aminophenols can generate methemoglobin. The mechanisms of action seems to be oxidation of the aminophenol to its corresponding quinoneimine, the latter oxidizing the hemoglobin Fe^{2+} to Fe^{3+} and being reduced to the aminophenol, setting up a catalytic cycle. Kiese and Weger[60] showed that, of a number of aminophenols investigated, DMAP generated therapeutic levels of methemoglobin most rapidly. Moreover, in a number of species—mice, dogs, rabbits, cynomolgus monkeys and humans[60,61]—DMAP acted faster in producing methemoglobin than sodium nitrite and other derivatives of aminophenol. In the short period of use of DMAP, there have been some case reports of unfavorable clinical experiences,[62–64] and the drug has not been widely adopted outside Germany. The main toxic effect of DMAP is the one it shares with other methemoglobin producers, namely the production of hypoxia. In experimental animals DMAP is nephrotoxic.[65] This would be unlikely to affect its use in humans, and the main question concerning DMAP is why it has proved unsatisfactory in clinical use, while sodium nitrite has been used for many years without major problems. A possible reason is that peak levels of methemoglobin generated by the recommended doses of the two compounds are very different, being much higher with DMAP.

DMAP is presented as 5-ml ampoules containing 250 mg DMAP, with 25 mg ascorbic acid and 10 mg disodium hydrogen phosphate ($Na_2HPO_4.12H_2O$). The recommended dose is 3.25 mg kg^{-1} intravenously. As with sodium nitrite, use of DMAP should be followed by sodium thiosulfate.

Aminophenones

Aminophenones, particularly 4-aminopropiophenone (*p*-aminopropiophenone, PAPP), have been studied in cyanide poisoning. However, because they require metabolic change to become active methemoglobin producers, it has generally been considered that aminophenones would constitute better prophylaxis than post-poisoning treatments. The mechanism of action of the proximate methemoglobin former, probably the *N*-hydroxyaminophenone, is rather different from that of the aminophenols.[65] The oxidation of Fe^{2+} to Fe^{3+} is accompanied by conversion of the hydroxyaminophenone to the nitroso derivative.[66,67] This is reduced, in the red cell, back to the hydroxyaminophenone by NADPH, thus setting up a catalytic circle.

COBALT COMPOUNDS

It has long been known that cyanides could form complexes of low toxicity with cobalt. On addition of potassium cyanide to cobalt compounds *in vitro*, a 5:1 cyanide–cobalt complex is formed.[68] However, during experiments *in vivo*, Evans[69] thought that each cobalt atom was antagonizing six molecules of cyanide, to form the cobalticyanide ion, and thence the cobaltocyanide ion. These complex cobalt–cyanide ions are of low toxicity, with LD$_{50}$s in the region of 1 g kg^{-1}.

Cobalt salts are somewhat toxic[70] and this fact militated against their use as cyanide antidotes for many years. However, in 1950 Muschett *et al.*[71] showed that hydroxocobalamin (vitamin B$_{12a}$), a complex cobalt-containing compound, could antagonize cyanide poisoning in experimental animals. Hydroxocobalamin (see below) is not a particularly convenient antidote, especially in a CW context. A number of investigators, including notably Paulet,[54,72–76] studied the antidotal efficacy and toxicity of various other cobalt compounds, both salts and organic complexes. On the basis of animal studies of both toxicity and efficacy against experimental cyanide poisoning, Paulet concluded that dicobalt edetate was the most satisfactory cobalt compound for the treatment of cyanide poisoning.

Dicobalt edetate

The usual preparation of dicobalt edetate is Kelocyanor (SERB, Paris). The 20-ml ampoules contain a solution of 0.196—0.240 g per 100 ml free cobalt and 1.35–1.65 g per 100 ml dicobalt edetate, as well as 4 g of glucose per ampoule. Although inorganic cobalt salts antagonize at a molar ratio of 6:1, dicobalt edetate only appears to antagonize at molar ratios of up to 2.[69] Kelocyanor has been widely adopted in Europe and a number of case reports attest to its efficacy. In industrial contexts, its rapidity of action has particularly impressed.[77] The main problems with dicobalt edetate seem to have occurred when dicobalt edetate has been administered to unpoisoned patients. These effects include urticaria, edema of the face, chest pains, dyspnea and hypotension, and may reflect the fact that dicobalt edetate has a higher LD_{50} in the presence of cyanide than in its absence. These effects can be minimized by injection of dextrose.

Dicobalt edetate has been compared in animal studies with a number of other cyanide antidotes and been found to be effective, possibly more so than the classical therapy and less so than 4-dimethylaminophenol (see below).

Hydroxocobalamin

Hydroxocobalamin, although an efficacious cyanide antidote, is inconvenient as presented in most preparations, which are designed for the treatment of pernicious anemia. Such preparations contain amounts of hydroxocobalamin that are negligible by comparison with those needed to antagonize meaningful quantities of HCN. Therefore, large volumes would have to be used. However, there has been much progress with this antidote in France (see Hall and Rumack[78] for a review).

COMPARISON OF CYANIDE ANTIDOTES

Many studies have been carried out comparing the main cyanide antidotal regimes (Table 5). Those carried out in rodents, where methemoglobin-producing antidotes were used, are difficult to interpret, as the much higher activity of erythrocytic methemoglobin reductase in rodents makes the results of studies difficult to extrapolate to humans. Furthermore, some of the studies cited in Table 5 made use of prophylactic protocols. Bearing in mind the difficulty of mimicking the situation in acute human poisoning in animals studied, the most that can be said is that 4-dimethylaminophenol is probably the most efficacious antidote. However, all the

Table 5. Comparative studies on cyanide antidotes

Antidotes compared	Model	Reference
Dicobalt edetate versus sodium nitrite	Dog	Paulet[74]
Dicobalt edetate versus sodium nitrite thiosulfate	Dog	Paulet[74]
Dicobalt edetate versus sodium nitrite	Mouse	Terzic and Milosevic[55]
Dicobalt edetate versus 4-dimethyl-aminophenol	Dog	Klimmek et al.[79]
Dicobalt edetate versus 4-dimethyl-aminophenol	Dog	Marrs et al.[80]
Dicobalt edetate versus sodium thiosulfate + rhodanese	Rabbit	Atkinson et al.[81]
Dicobalt edetate versus other cobalt compounds	Mouse/rabbit	Evans[69]
Sodium nitrite versus 4-dimethyl-aminophenol	Cat	Schwarzkopf and Friedberg[82]
Sodium nitrite versus 4-dimethyl-aminophenol	Mouse	Kruszyna et al.[83]

main clinically used antidotes seem capable of resuscitating acutely poisoned experimental animals and patients.

TREATMENT OF HYDROGEN CYANIDE POISONING UNDER BATTLEFIELD CONDITIONS

It will have been noted that with the exception of the perhaps not very effective inhalation of amyl nitrite, all cyanide antidotes have to be administered intravenously and generally in large (>10 ml) volumes. Troops affected by HCN could not be expected to administer antidotes in this way to themselves, and nor is it likely that untrained colleagues would be able to undertake this task. On a battlefield the problems posed by giving an intravenous injection, whilst both the attendant and the casualty are wearing full chemical protective equipment, would be overwhelming: exposure of a suitable vein will itself be difficult, though not dangerous if it is known that the attack has consisted of HCN vapor only: HCN vapor is not absorbed across the skin. At a first aid post it might be expected that cyanide antidotes could be administered.

PROPHYLAXIS OF CYANIDE POISONING

Because of the rapidity with which HCN poisoning must be treated for there to be any realistic prospect of success, prophylaxis has been studied by a number of workers. Bright[84] reviewed this topic and concluded that an orally active drug, with a long duration of activity and low toxicity, would be required. Some studies were carried out on DMAP, but most work has been undertaken using PAPP. Studies in animals showed that a 12–15% methemoglobinemia generated by DMAP was effective against the lethal effects in dogs of 2 × LD$_{50}$ HCN[85] and that a similar methemoglobinemia generated by PAPP was effective against the sublethal effects of a dose of about the LD$_{50}$ of HCN.[84] Because the duration of the therapeutic methemoglobinemia produced by PAPP is not much more than 2 h, studies were carried out using aminophenones with longer aliphatic chains. Such compounds, particularly 4-aminooctanoylphenone, produced therapeutic methemoglobinemia for a longer duration, which would allow much less frequent administration. Certain other long-acting methemoglobin formers, such as the 8-aminoquinoline derivatives studied by Steinhaus et al.,[86] might also be useful in HCN prophylaxis.

OXYGEN IN CYANIDE POISONING

For many years it was believed that oxygen had no role in the treatment of poisoning by cyanides. The rationale for this belief was that the blood was fully oxygenated in cyanide poisoning and it was utilization that was arrested. However, a number of studies, for example those of Way,[87] and Sheehy and Way,[88] have shown that oxygen enhances the antidotal effects of the classical cyanide antidotes. The mechanism may be by enhancing detoxication or elimination of cyanide, as the inhibition of cytochrome oxidase by cyanide is unaffected by oxygen.[89]

REFERENCES

1. Guatelli MA (1964) The toxicology of cyanides. In: *Methods in Forensic Sciences*, Vol. 3 (AS Curry, ed.), pp. 233–265. New York: Academic Press.
2. Isom GE and Way JL (1984) Effects of oxygen on antagonism of cyanide intoxication: cytochrome oxidase in vitro. *Toxicol Appl Pharmacol*, **74**, 57–62.
3. Katsumata Y, Sato K, Oya M et al. (1980) Kinetic analysis of the shift of aerobic to anaerobic metabolism in rats during acute cyanide poisoning. *Life Sci*, **27**, 1509–1512.
4. Johnson JD, Meisenheimer TL and Isom GE (1986) Cyanide-induced neurotoxicity; role of neuronal calcium. *Toxicol Appl Pharmacol*, **84**, 464–469.
5. Maduh EU, Turek JJ, Borowitz JL et al. (1990) Calcium mediation of morphological changes in neuronal cells. *Toxicol Appl Pharmacol*, **103**, 214–221.
6. McNamara BP (1976) Estimates of the toxicity of hydrocyanic acid vapors in man. Washington DC: US Department of Defense.
7. Barcroft J (1931) The toxicity of atmospheres containing hydrocyanic acid gas. *J Hygiene*, **31**, 1–34.
8. Marrs TC (1988) Antidotal treatment of acute cyanide poisoning. *Adverse Drug React Acute Pois Rev*, **4**, 179–206.
9. Bright JE and Marrs TC (1988) The pharmacokinetics of intravenous potassium cyanide. *Human Toxicol*, **7**, 183–186.
10. Soine WH, Brady KT, Balster RL and Underwood JQ (1980) Chemical and behavioral studies of 1-piperidinocyclohexanecarbonitrile (PCC): evidence for cyanide as the toxic component. *Res Commun Chem Pathol Pharmacol*, **30**, 59–70.

11. Vedder EB (1925) *The Medical Aspects of Chemical Warfare*, Baltimore: Williams and Wilkins.

12. Peters CG, Mundy JVB and Rayner PR (1982) Acute cyanide poisoning: the treatment of a suicide attempt. *Anaesthesia*, **37**, 582–586.

13. Finelli PF (1981) Changes in the basal ganglia following cyanide poisoning. *J Computer Assisted Tomogr*, **5**, 755–756.

14. Uitti RJ, Rajput AH, Ashenhurst EM and Rozdilsky B (1985) Cyanide-induced parkinsonism: a clinicopathologic report. *Neurology*, **35**, 921–925.

15. Marrs TC and Bright JE (1985) Protection by p-aminopropiophenone against cyanide-induced sublethal effects. *J Toxicol Clin Toxicol*, **23**, 462–463.

16. D'Mello GD (1987) Neuropathological and behavioural sequelae of acute cyanide toxicosis in animal species. In: *Clinical and Experimental Toxicology of Cyanides* (B Ballantyne and TC Marrs, eds), pp. 156–183. Bristol: John Wright.

17. Bass NH (1968) Pathogenesis of myelin lesions in experimental cyanide encephalopathy. *Neurology*, **18**, 167–177.

18. Levine S and Stypulkowski W (1959) Experimental cyanide encephalopathy. *Arch Pathol*, **67**, 306–323.

19. Haymaker W, Ginzler AM and Ferguson RL (1952) Residual neuropathological effects of cyanide poisoning. *Mil Surgeon*, **111**, 231–246.

20. Hertting G, Kraupp O, Schnetz E and Wuketich S (1960) Untersuchungen über die Folgen einer chronischen Verabreichung akut toxischer Dosen von Natriumcyanid an Hunden. *Acta Pharmacol Toxicol*, **17**, 27–43.

21. Funata N, Song S-Y, Okeda R *et al.* (1984) A study of experimental cyanide encephalopathy in the acute phase—physiological and neurological correlation. *Acta Neuropathol (Berlin)*, **64**, 99–107.

22. Wilson J (1987) Cyanide in human disease. In: *Clinical and Experimental Toxicology of Cyanides* (B Ballantyne and TC Marrs, eds), pp. 292–311. Bristol: John Wright.

23. Ballantyne B and Marrs TC (1987) Post-mortem features and criteria for the diagnosis of acute lethal cyanide poisoning. In: *Clinical and Experimental Toxicology of Cyanides* (B Ballantyne and TC Marrs, eds), pp. 217–247. Bristol, John Wright.

24. Varnell RM, Stimac GK and Fligner CL (1987) CT diagnosis of toxic brain injury in cyanide poisoning: considerations in forensic medicine. *Am J Neuroradiol*, **8**, 1063–1066.

25. Ballantyne B, Bright JE and Williams P (1974) The post-mortem rate of transformation of cyanide. *Forensic Sci*, **3**, 71–76.

26. Way JL, Holmes R and Way JL (1985) Cyanide antagonism with mercaptopyruvate. *Fed Proc*, **44**, 718.

27. Baskin SI and Kirkby SD (1990) The effect of sodium tetrathionate on cyanide conversion of thiocyanate by enzymatic and non-enzymatic mechanisms. *J Appl Toxicol*, **10**, 379–382.

28. Smith RP (1969) Cobalt salts: effects in cyanide and sulfide poisoning and on methemoglobinomia. *Toxicol Appl Pharmacol*, **15**, 505–516.

29. Jianyao M, Yu W and Laifa Q (1987) Antidotal effect of intramuscularly administered sodium cobaltinitrite on cyanide poisoning. *F Med Cell PLA*, **2**, 301–305.

30. Bhattacharya R, Jeevaratnam K, Raza SK and Das Gupta S (1993) Protection against cyanide poisoning by co-administration of sodium nitrite and hydroxylamine in rats. *Human Exp Toxicol*, **12**, 33–36.

31. Schwartz C, Morgan RL, Way LM and Way JL (1979) Antagonism of cyanide intoxication with sodium pyruvate. *Toxicol Appl Pharmacol*, **50**, 437–441.

32. Keniston RL, Calbellon S and Yarborough KS (1987) Pyridoxal 5'-phosphate as an antidote for cyanide, spermine, gentomycin and dopamine toxicity: an *in vivo* rat study. *Toxicol Appl Pharmacol*, **88**, 433–441.

33. Way JL and Burrows G (1976) Cyanide intoxication: protection with chlorpromazine. *Toxicol Appl Pharmacol*, **36**, 93–97.

34. Leung P, Sylvester DM, Chiou F *et al.* (1984) Effect of naloxone HCl on cyanide intoxication. *Fed Proc*, **43**, 545.

35. Rump S and Edelwejn Z (1968) Effects of centrophenoxone on electrical activity of the rabbit brain in cyanide intoxication. *Int J Neuropharmacol*, **7**, 103–113.

36. Burrows GE and Way JL (1976) Antagonism of cyanide toxicity with phenoxybenzamine. *Fed Proc*, **35**, 533.

37. Vick JH and Frochlich HL (1985) Studies of cyanide poisoning. *Arch Int Pharmacodyn*, **273**, 314–322.

38. Isom GE and Johnson JD (1987) Sulphur donors in cyanide intoxication In: *Clinical and Experimental Toxicology of Cyanides* (B Ballantyne and TC Marrs, eds), pp. 413–426. Bristol: John Wright.

39. Sylvester DM, Hayton WL, Schneiderhan W and Kiese M (1983) Effects of thiosulfate on cyanide pharmacokinetics in dogs. *Toxicol Appl Pharmacol*, **69**, 265–271.

40. Christel D, Eyer P, Hegemann M *et al.* (1977) Pharmacokinetics of cyanide poisoning in dogs, and the effect of 4-dimethylaminophenol or thiosulfate. *Arch Toxicol*, **38**, 177–189.

41. Clemedson CJ, Hultman HI and Sörbo B (1954) The antidote effect of some sulfur compounds in experimental cyanide poisoning. *Acta Physiol Scand*, **32**, 245–251.

42. Frankenberg L (1980) Enzyme therapy in cyanide poisoning: effect of rhodanese and sulfur compounds. *Arch Toxicol*, **45**, 315–323.

43. Leung P, Davis RW, Yao CC *et al.* (1984) Rhodanese and sodium thiosulfate encapsulated in mouse carrier erythrocytes. II *In vivo* survivability and alterations in physiologic and morphologic characteristics. *Fund Appl Toxicol*, **16**, 559–566.

44. Hambright P (1986) Anti-cyanide drugs. US Department of Defense: Annual Summary Report, US Army Medical Research and Development Command, Fort Detrick, Maryland 21701 USA. Unclassified Report.

45. Ten Eyck RP, Schaerdel AD and Ottinger WE (1985) Stroma-free methemoglobin solution: an effective antidote for acute cyanide poisoning. *Am J Emerg Med*, **3**, 519–523.

46. Boswell GW, Brooks DE, Murray AJ *et al.* (1988) Exogenous methemoglobin as a cyanide antidote in rats. *Pharmacol Res*, **5**, 749–752.

47. Pedigo LG (1888) Antagonism between amyl nitrite and prussic acid. *Trans Med Soc Virginia*, **19**, 124–131.

48. Bastian G and Mercker H (1959) Zur der Frage der Zweckmäßigkeit der Inhalation von Amylnitrit in der Behandlung der Cyanidvergiftung. *Naunyn-Schmiedebergs Arch Exp Pathol Toxikol*, **237**, 285–295.

49. Chen KK, Rose CL and Clowes GHA (1933) Amyl nitrite and cyanide poisoning. *JAMA*, **100**, 1920–1922.

50. Paulet G (1954) Sur la valeur du nitrite d'amyle dans le traitement de l'intoxication cyanhydrique. *CR Soc Biol*, **148**, 1009–1014.

51. Pierce JMT and Nielsen MS (1989) Acute acquired methaemoglobinaemia after amyl nitrate poisoning. *Br Med J*, **298**, 1566.

52. Hug E (1933) Acción del nitrito de sodio y del hiposulfito de sodio en el tratamiento de la intoxicación provocada por el cianuro de potasio en el conejo. *Rev Soc Argentinians Biol*, **9**, 91–97.

53. Chen KK, Rose CL and Clowes GHA (1933) Methylene blue, nitrites and sodium thiosulfate against cyanide poisoning. *Proc Soc Exp Biol Med*, **31**, 250–252.

54. Paulet G (1961) Nouvelles perspectives dans le traitement de l'intoxication cyanhydrique. *Arch Mal Prof*, **22**, 120–127.

55. Terzic M and Milosevic M (1963) Action protectrice de l'éthylène-diamine-tétra-acétate-dicobaltique dans l'intoxication cyanée. *Thérapie*, **18**, 55–61.

56. Holmes RK and Way JL (1982) Mechanism of cyanide antagonism by sodium nitrite. *Pharmacologist*, **24**, 182.

57. Berlin CM (1970) The treatment of cyanide poisoning in children. *Pediatrics*, **46**, 793–796.

58. Shuval HI and Kruener N (1972) Epidemiological and toxicological aspects of nitrates and nitrites in the environment. *Am J Publ Hlth*, **161**, 163–168.

59. Metcalf WK (1961) Experimental oxidation of haemoglobin and its relation to growth rates in rats. *Nature*, **190**, 543–544.

60. Kiese M and Weger N (1969) Formation of ferrihaemoglobin with aminophenols in the human for the treatment of cyanide poisoning. *Eur J Pharmacol*, **7**, 97–105.

61. Hawkins SF, Groff WA, Johnson RP *et al.* (1981) Comparison of the *in vivo* formation of methemoglobin by 4-dimethyl aminophenol and sodium nitrite in the cynomolgus monkey. *Fed Proc*, **40**, 718.

62. van Dijk A, Douze JMC, van Heijst ANP and Glerum J (1986) Clinical evaluation of the cyanide antidote 4-DMP. In: *Proceedings of the IIIrd World Congress of the World Federation of Associations of Clinical Toxicology and Poisons Control Centers and the XIIth International Congress of the European Association of Poisons Control Centres*, p. 49. Brussels, 27–30 August 1986.

63. van Dijk A, Glerum JH, van Heijst ANP and Douze JMC (1987) Clinical evaluation of the cyanide antagonist 4-DMAP in a lethal cyanide poisoning case. *Vet Hum Toxicol*, **29** (Suppl. 2), 38–39.

64. van Heijst ANP, Douze JMC, van Kesteren RG *et al.* Therapeutic problems in cyanide poisoning. *Clin Toxicol*, **25**, 383–398.

65. Szinicz LL (1979) Nephrotoxicität von Aminophenolen: Wirkung von 4-Dimethyl-aminophenol auf isolierte Nierentubuli von Ratten. *Fortschr Med*, **46**, 1206–1208.

66. Graffe W, Kiese M and Rauscher E (1964) The formation *in vivo* of p-hydroxylamino-propiophenone from p-aminopropiophenone and its action *in vivo* and *in vitro*. *Naunyn-Schmiedebergs Arch Exp Pathol Pharmacol*, **249**, 168–175.

67. Marrs TC, Inns RH, Bright JE and Wood SG (1991) The formation of methaemoglobin by 4-aminopropiophenone (PAPP) and 4-(N-hydroxy)aminopropiophenone. *Hum Exp Toxicol*, **10**, 183–188.

68. Cotton FA and Wilkinson G (1966) *Advanced Inorganic Chemistry*, 2nd edn. New York and London: Interscience.

69. Evans CL (1964) Cobalt compounds as antidotes for hydrocyanic acid. *Br J Pharmacol*, **23**, 455–475.

70. Speijers GJA, Krajnc EI, Berkvens JM and van Lolgten MJ (1982) Acute oral toxicity of inorganic cobalt compounds in rats. *Food Chem Toxicol*, **20**, 311–314.

71. Muschett CW, Kelly KL, Boxer GE and Rickards (1952) Antidotal efficacy of vitamin B12a (Hydroxo-cobalamin) in experimental cyanide poisoning. *Proc Soc Exp Biol (New York)*, **81**, 234–237.

72. Paulet G (1957) Valeur des sels organiques du cobalt dans le traitement de l'intoxication cyanhydrique. *CR Soc Biol*, **151**, 1932–1935.

73. Paulet G (1958) L'intoxication cyanhydrique et chélates de cobalt. *J Physiol (Paris)*, **50**, 438–442.

74. Paulet G (1960) *L'intoxication cyanhydrique et son traitement*. Paris: Masson SA.

75. Paulet G (1960) Les chélates de cobalt dans le traitement de l'intoxication cyanhydrique. *Path Biol*, **8**, 255–266.

76. Paulet G (1965) Au sujet du traitement de l'intoxication cyanhydrique par les chélates de cobalt. *Urgence*, **11**, 611–613.

77. Bryson DD (1987) Acute industrial cyanide intoxication and its treatment. In: *Clinical and Experimental Toxicology of Cyanides* (B Ballantyne and TC Marrs, eds), pp. 348–358. Bristol: John Wright.

78. Hall HH and Rumack BH (1987) Hydroxocobalamin/sodium thiosulfate as a cyanide antidote. *F Emerg Med*, **5**, 115–121.

79. Klimmek R, Fladerer H and Weger N (1979) Circulation, respiration, and blood

homeostasis in cyanide poisoned dogs after treatment with 4-dimethylaminophenol or cobalt compounds. *Arch Toxicol*, **43**, 121–133.

80. Marrs TC, Swanston DW and Bright JE (1985) 4-Dimethyl aminophenol and dicobaltedetate (Kelocyanor) in the treatment of experimental cyanide poisoning. *Hum Toxicol*, **4**, 541–600.

81. Atkinson A, Rutter DA and Sergeant K (1974) Enzyme antidote for experimental cyanide poisoning. *Lancet*, **II**, 1446.

82. Schwarzkopf HA and Friedberg KD (1971) Zur Beurteilung der Blausäure-Antidote. *Arch Toxikol*, **27**, 111–123.

83. Kruszyna R, Kruszyna S and Smith RP (1982) Comparison of hydroxylamine, 4-dimethylaminophenol and nitrite protection against cyanide poisoning in mice. *Arch Toxicol*, **49**, 191–202.

84. Bright JE (1987) A prophylaxis for cyanide poisoning In: *Clinical and Experimental Toxicology of Cyanides* (B Ballantyne and TC Marrs, eds), pp. 359–382. Bristol: John Wright.

85. Marrs TC, Bright JE and Swanston DW (1982) The effect of prior treatment with 4-dimethylaminophenol (DMAP) on animals experimentally poisoned with hydrogen cyanide. *Arch Toxicol*, **51**, 247–253.

86. Steinhaus RK, Baskin SI, Clark JH and Kirby SD (1990) Formation of methemoglobin and metmyoglobin using 8-aminoquinoline derivatives or sodium nitrite and subsequent reaction with cyanide. *J Appl Toxicol*, **10**, 345–351.

87. Way JL (1984) Cyanide intoxication and its mechanism of antagonism. *Ann Ther Pharmacol Toxicol*, **24**, 451–481.

88. Sheehy M and Way JL (1968) Effect of oxygen on cyanide intoxication III mithridate. *J Pharmacol Ther*, **161**, 163–168.

89. Way JL, Gibbon SL and Sheehy M (1966) Effect of oxygen on cyanide intoxication 1. Prophylactic protection. *J Pharmacol Exp Ther*, **153**, 381–385.

RIOT-CONTROL AGENTS

Riot-control agents are not really chemical warfare agents. Their effect, as intended, is not to kill or even seriously injure, but simply to incapacitate. The main effect of all riot-control agents is to incapacitate by irritating the skin and mucous membranes. The first was ethyl bromoacetate, used in Paris in 1912. The three most frequently used ones are DM, CN and CS (Table 1). CR has been developed most recently but has rarely been used. There is a surprising amount of toxicological data on all four agents, especially CS.

2-CHLOROBENZILIDENE MALONONITRILE (CS)

CS is by far the most important of the riot-control agents. Part 1 of the Himsworth report into the use of CS in Derry (Northern Ireland) stated that riot-control agents should be viewed 'more akin to that from which we regard the effects of a new drug than to that from which we might regard a weapon'.[1] As a result, as much is known of the toxicity of CS as for many regulated chemicals such as pesticides or drugs.

CS is a white crystalline solid, first synthesized by Corson and Staughton in 1928. Dispersed as a smoke or fog, CS has achieved use as a riot-control agent on account of its potent sensory irritant effects. Hand-held devices, where CS is dispersed as an aerosol, are available, but these are illegal in the UK.

CS is an SN_2-type alkylating agent (substitution nucleophilic second order), as are most riot-control agents, with the important exception of CR (dibenz [b,f]-1,4-oxazepine). In the case of these SN_2-type alkylating agents such as CS, CN and CA (α-bromobenzalcyanide), the strong electron-pulling groups, chlorine or bromine, together with the nitrile radical, render the benzyl carbon atom relatively electropositive.[2]

Table 1. Riot-control agents

Code	Chemical name
DM	10-Chloro-5,10-dihydrophenarsazine
CN	2-Chloroacetophenone
CS	2-Chlorobenzilidene malononitrile
CR	Dibenz(b.f.)-1:4-oxazepine

Absorption, distribution and metabolism

In the circumstances in which it is usually used, CS is predominantly a respiratory and to some extent a percutaneous hazard. However, the gastrointestinal route must be considered in relation to swallowed nasal secretion.

ABSORPTION AND METABOLISM AFTER INHALATION

Several studies have been undertaken into the absorption and metabolism of CS after inhalation exposure. Leadbeater[3] showed that rats exposed to CS aerosols at concentrations of 14–245 mg m^{-3} for 5 min absorbed measurable quantities of the compound. Both CS and a reduction product, 2-chlorobenzyl malononitrile, were detected in the blood. In rats exposed to CS concentrations greater than 100 mg m^{-3}, 2-chlorobenzaldehyde was also detected. In similar studies in cats the same three compounds (CS, 2-chlorobenzaldehyde and 2-chlorobenzyl malononitrile) were detected in the blood.

METABOLIC STUDIES BY ROUTES OTHER THAN INHALATION

When CS was administered by gavage to rats, it was only detected in the blood after very high doses. 2-Chlorobenzaldehyde and 2-chlorobenzyl malononitrile were present after much lower doses. The same substances were found in cats after intragastric administration of CS but at much lower CS doses.[3] CS disappears from the circulation very rapidly,[3] as do chlorobenzyl malononitrile and 2-chlorobenzaldehyde, approximating to first-order kinetics up to 525 nmol kg^{-1}. The half-lives estimated by Leadbeater after intra-arterial injection into cats were 5.5 s for CS, 9.5 s for chlorobenzyl malononitrile and 4.5 s for 2-chlorobenzaldehyde. *In vitro* in cat blood, the half-life of 2-chlorobenzyl malononitrile is markedly longer (470 s). Rat blood appeared to break down CS metabolites more rapidly than cat blood. The 2-chlorobenzaldehyde is further metabolized to 2-chlorobenzoic acid, the main metabolite detectable in rat urine being 2-chlorohippuric acid.[2,4] Other metabolites that have been observed include 2-chlorobenzyl glucopyranosuric acid, 2-chlorobenzyl cysteine, 2-chlorobenzoic acid, 2-chlorophenyl acetylglycine and 2-chlorobenzyl-mercapturic acid.[4,5]

There appear to be significant species differences in urinary metabolites observed. Chassaud[6] studied the glutathione *S*-alkenetransferases of the livers of various mammalian species with respect to metabolism of CS: a number of interesting differences were found between the species studied, including an absence of activity in rabbit liver. In fact, Rietveld *et al.*[5] have shown that CS injected intraperitoneally into rats causes the excretion of 2-chlorobenzylmercapturic acid (*N*-acetyl-*S*-(2-chlorobenzyl)-L-cysteine). Their data led them to believe that this mercapturic acid resulted from a reaction with 2-chlorobenzaldehyde rather than a direct addition of glutathione to CS.

CS CYANOGENESIS

According to Cuccinell et al.[2] CS reacts very rapidly with plasma protein, probably generating covalent addition compounds. In water CS is rapidly hydrolysed to 2-chlorobenzaldehyde and malononitrile, the latter giving rise to cyanide and thiocyanate. Free cyanide is present in animals after intravenous CS, and thiocyanate was identified by Brewster et al.[4] in the urine of rats after intraperitoneal and gavage administration. Likewise, thiocyanate was observed in the urine of mice after both parenteral and inhalation administration by Frankenberg and Sörbo.[7] Moreover, in this study the cyanide antidote sodium thiosulphate decreased the toxicity of CS. However, in dogs cyanogenesis was not observed even after lethal doses of aerosol.[2] Comparison of the molar lethal doses of CS and cyanide suggest that only one CN group is produced per mole of CS.

METABOLIC STUDIES IN HUMANS

Leadbeater[3] exposed six male volunteers to CS at concentrations of 0.5–1.5 mg m^{-3} for 90 min. Neither CS nor 2-chlorobenzaldehyde was detected in the blood of those persons, and only in one was a trace of 2-chlorobenzyl malononitrile detected.

TOXICOLOGY

ACUTE TOXICITY—SMOKE

On the basis of experimental determinations of the lethal dose in five different species, Punte et al.[8] concluded that CS had a higher safety ratio (irritant concentration compared with lethal concentration) than any other sensory irritant of its type. Pyrotechnically generated CS did not kill animals after exposure for 30 min to concentrations 100 times or more than those expected to be produced by functioning CS grenades in the open air.

Ballantyne and Callaway[9] investigated the toxicity of pyrotechnically generated CS to guinea pigs, rats, rabbits and mice (Table 2). The lungs of decedents were oedematous and congested with multiple haemorrhages. The tracheas and bronchi contained excessive mucus. On microscopic examination haemorrhagic atelectasis was seen. There was evidence of circulatory failure. Similar changes were also seen in the decedents from experiments in which the same species were exposed to similar doses of CS over a longer time. Exposure of rats to very large single doses of CS (30 000–90 000 mg min m^{-3}) showed that CS smoke gave rise to congestion and severe capillary damage, but a time-course study showed that the induced damage as revealed by electron microscopy was only transient.[10]

Ballantyne and Callaway[9] exposed rats and hamsters to doses of CS (750 mg m^{-3} for 30 min, 480 mg m^{-3} for 60 min and 150 mg m^{-3} for 120 min) and sacrificed the animals at intervals thereafter. At the highest concentration no deaths occurred. In sacrificed animals, minimal lung pathology was observed in hamsters sacrificed at 1 day; little of note was seen in rats at that time or in either species sacrificed at 10 or 28

Table 2. Acute single-dose toxicity of CS smoke

	LCt_{50} with 95% confidence limits (mg min m^{-3})	
Guinea pig	35 800	(24 200–50 500)
Rabbit	63 600	(45 800–89 200)
Rat	69 800	(55 600–90 000)
Mouse	70 900	(56 600–91 800)

Data from Ballantyne and Callaway.[9]

days. After 480 mg m^{-3} for 60 min, more hamsters died than rats, mostly with lung lesions. An interesting finding in both species was tubular necrosis in the kidneys; 150 mg m^{-3} for 120 min was less toxic, and sacrificed animals showed few abnormalities.

CS AEROSOLS

Table 3 shows the acute LCt_{50} for CS aerosol in a number of species. In the cases of the guinea pig and rat it is higher than the LCt_{50} for the smoke; in the mouse it is somewhat lower. Histological examination of decedents from that study showed similar changes to those seen after exposure to the smoke. Animals surveyed after 14 days appeared normal.[11]

ACUTE TOXICITY OF CS BY ROUTES OTHER THAN INHALATION

The acute toxicity of CS by routes other than inhalation was investigated by Ballantyne and Swanston[11] (Table 4). The oral toxicity is lower than that of CN in rats, rabbits and guinea pigs, the difference being most notable in rats, where it is about 1 g kg^{-1} as against 127 mg kg^{-1} for CN. CS is also less toxic by the intraperitoneal route in male rats and female guinea pigs. It is noteworthy, however, in the case of female rabbits, male mice and female rats that CS is more toxic than CN.

Table 3. Acute single-dose toxicity of CS aerosol

	LCt_{50} with 95% confidence limits (mg min m^{-3})	
Guinea pig (female)	67 200	(59 200–78 450)
Rabbit (female)	54 090	(42 630–70 400)
Rat (male)	88 480	(77 370–98 520)
Mouse (male)	50 010	(42 750–60 220)

Data from Ballantyne and Swanston.[11]

Table 4. Toxicity of CS by routes other than inhalation

Route	Species	LD_{50} (mg kg^{-1})	95% confidence limits
IV	Rabbit (female)	27	24–31
	Mouse (male)	48	43–56
	Rat (female)	28	25–30
IP	Rat (male)	48	43–54
	Guinea pig (female)	73	62–79
Oral	Rat (female)	1284	1134–1531
	Rat (male)	1366	1184–1779
	Guinea pig (female)	212	190–244
	Rabbit (male)	231	186–493
	Rabbit (female)	143	61–236

Data from Ballantyne and Swanston.[11]

MECHANISM OF THE ACUTE TOXICITY OF CS

Many of the changes seen in the lungs with CS smoke are similar in quality to those produced by other irritant smokes. The lethality of CS is probably dependent on two main factors:[11] its alkylating properties and its cyanogenic potential. On the first point, CS reacts with glutathione,[2,6] and also lipoic acid and cysteine,[2] and Ballantyne and Swanston state that the alkylating properties of the molecule are major determinants of the toxicity of CS after intravenous administration. There is also evidence that cyanide contributes to the toxicity of CS (see above).

LONG-TERM TOXICITY OF CS

Marrs *et al.*[12] exposed mice, rats and guinea pigs to CS for 1 h per day, 5 days per week, for up to 120 days. Animals were then observed for 6 months and the survivors were sacrificed. Exposure concentrations were approximately 0.3, 30 and 200 μg l^{-1}. Exposure of the highest group was stopped after 3–5 exposures, because of high mortality. A few pathological changes were observed that showed a relationship with exposure, mostly chronic inflammatory changes in the lungs, especially in the guinea pigs. There was no evidence of a tumorigenic response to CS, although the study was too short to exclude the possibility that CS had tumorigenic potential. The authors concluded that 30 μg l^{-1} could be considered a no-adverse-effect concentration for CS. Marrs *et al.*[13] exposed rats and hamsters to a single dose of CS of either 28 800 mg min m^{-3} or 18 000 mg min m^{-3}, the animals being observed for up to 32 months. The procedure had no effect on survival and no other test-material-related effects were observed.

EMBRYOTOXICITY

The embryotoxicity of CS was studied in Porton rats and New Zealand White rabbits by Upshall.[14] Rats and rabbits were exposed by inhalation to the aerosol (1–2 μm mass median aerodynamic diameter (mad)) on days 6–15 and days 6–18 of pregnancy at concentrations of 6, 20 or 60 mg m^{-3} for 5 min per day. Additionally, rats were exposed by the intraperitoneal route to CS in PEG 300 on days 6, 8, 10, 12 or 14 of pregnancy. CS was neither embryolethal nor teratogenic.

MUTAGENICITY OF CS

Von Däniken et al.[15] found a weak mutagenic effect in the Ames test with strain TA 100 but not TA 1535, 1537, 1538 or 98. The effect in TA 100 was weak and only observed without preincubation with S9. High doses of CS (up to 100 and 2000 μg per plate) were bacteriotoxic. CS showed little evidence of binding to DNA in an in vivo assay in rats but bound strongly to nuclear proteins. It was to that effect that von Däniken et al. ascribed the cytotoxic effects of CS. CS was again tested for mutagenic potential in the Ames test, but using Salmonella typhimurium TA 100 only;[5] CS was not mutagenic but it was bacteriotoxic in the assay. The CS putative metabolites 2-chlorobenzaldehyde, 2-chlorobenzyl alcohol, 2-chlorobenzyl sulphate, malononitrile and sodium cyanide were also tested in the Ames test using TA 100. All were negative. A further Ames test was carried out using Salmonella typhimurium strains TA 97a, TA 98, TA 100, TA 102 and TA 104; a mutagenic response was not observed in any strain, with or without S9.[16] CS gave small but significant responses in the L5178Y TK^{+-} mouse lymphoma cell forward mutation assay, without S9.[17] Schmid et al.[18] reported that exposure of V79 Chinese hamster ovary cells to CS caused a dose-dependent increase in the frequency of spindle disturbances and they therefore suggested that CS might induce aneuploidy in mammals. A study in vivo was carried out by Wild et al.[19] in Drosophila for the frequency of X-linked recessive mutations, and both this and a micronucleus test in mice was negative. Thus von Däniken's weak positive in a single strain has not been replicated by other workers. Although there is evidence for mutagenic activity in a mammalian cell system, there is no evidence of mutagenic activity in vivo.

OTHER ANIMAL STUDIES

CS is reported to inhibit adrenal steroidogenesis.[20]

HUMAN STUDIES AND REPORTS

Contact dermatitis was reported in 25/28 workers in a US chemical plant manufacturing CS.[21] A case of allergic contact dermatitis was reported by Fuchs and Ippen[22] from Germany.

A study of the effect of particle size on human reactions to CS was carried out by Owens and Punte.[23] They showed that a large-particle aerosol (60 μm) had less effect upon the respiratory system than a small-particle aerosol (1 μm). Large particles predominantly produced eye irritation. A volunteer study in 35 men was carried out by Beswick et al.[24] Tolerance to the effects of CS was noted and no abnormality was seen in ECG, respiratory function test or biochemical and haematological investigations.

Clinical signs and symptoms observed included stinging and watering of the eyes and nose, mouth and throat irritation, tightness of the chest and cough. There was a rise in blood pressure which was attributed to the discomfort. A case report by Park and Giammona[25] records prolonged non-lethal exposure of an infant which led to a secondary lung infection.

Treatment

Treatment is often not necessary: where it is, only aeration and irrigation are necessary. Irrigation of the eyes may be needed, where they have been severely contaminated, while areas of extensive skin contamination should be washed with copious amounts of water.[26] Protection against CS can be achieved by use of a respirator, while the eyes alone can be protected by soft contact lenses.[27]

Safety in use

CS is of moderate acute toxicity and is non-teratogenic. There is some evidence for mutagenicity *in vitro*, but none for activity *in vivo*. A 120-day repeated-dose study in three species gave a no adverse effect level (NOAEL) of 30 μg l^{-1}. Ballantyne[28] gave the TC_{50} (concentration intolerable to 50% of the population) as 3.6 μg l^{-1}. The ratio between the acute LC_{50} in animals and this is enormous, and there is an approximately 10-fold ratio between the IC_{50} and the repeated-dose NEL. Thus even repeated exposure to CS is unlikely to give rise to harm.

CN

CN aerosol is less effective than CS in its irritant effect, both upon the eye and the respiratory tract. It is of a similar order of toxicity as CS by the intravenous, intraperitoneal and oral routes. In most studies[28] CN is more toxic by inhalation than CS. CN can produce corneal epithelial damage as well as chemosis. Estimates of the LCt_{50} for humans of about 7000 mg min m^{-3}[29] are lower than those for CS (25 000–100 000 mg min m^{-3}).[30] Thus from the point of view of both safety and efficacy, CS seems preferable to CN.

CR

CR is slightly more effective than CS as an irritant and less toxic by all routes, particularly inhalation. CR differs from CS in not being an SN_2 alkylating agent and in its stability to hydrolysis. It has not been used for riot control.

REFERENCES

1. Himsworth H (1969) Report of the enquiry into the medical and toxicological aspects of CS (orthochlorobenzylidene malononitrile). Part 1, Command 4173. London: HMSO.
2. Cuccinell SA, Swentzel KC, Biskup R et al. (1971) Biochemical interactions and metabolic fate of riot control agents. Fed Proc, 30, 86–91.
3. Leadbeater L (1973) The absorption of ortho-chlorobenzylidenemalononitrile (CS) by the respiratory tract. Toxicol Appl Pharmacol, 25, 101–110.
4. Brewster K, Harrison JM, Leadbeater L et al. (1987). The fate of 2-chlorobenzylidene malononitrile (CS) in rats. Xenobiotica, 17, 911–924.
5. Rietveld EC, Delbressine LPC, Waegemaekers THJM and Seutter-Berlage F (1983) 2-Chlorobenzylmercapturic acid, a metabolite of the riot control agent, 2-chlorobenzylidene malononitrile (CS) in the rat. Arch Toxicol, 54, 139–144.
6. Chassaud L (1973) Distribution of enzymes that catalyse reactions of glutathione with αβ-unsaturated compounds. Biochem J, 131, 765–769.
7. Frankenberg L and Sörbo B (1973) Formation of cyanide from o-chlorobenzilidene malononitrile and its toxicological significance. Arch Toxicol, 31, 99–108.
8. Punte CL, Weimer JT, Ballard TA and Wilding JL (1962) Toxicologic studies on o-chlorobenzylidene malononitrile. Toxicol Appl Pharmacol, 4, 656.
9. Ballantyne B and Callaway S (1972) Inhalation toxicology and pathology of animals exposed to o-chlorobenzylidene malononitrile (CS). Med Sci Law, 12, 43–65.
10. Colgrave HF and Creasey JM (1975) Ultrastructure of rat lungs following exposure to o-chlorobenzylidene malononitrile (CS). Med Sci Law, 15, 187–197.
11. Ballantyne B and Swanston DW (1978) The comparative acute mammalian toxicity of 1-chloroacetophenone (CN) and 2-chlorobenzylidene malononitrile (CS). Arch Toxicol, 40, 75–95.
12. Marrs TC, Colgrave HF, Cross NL et al. (1983) A repeated dose study of the toxicity of inhaled 2-chlorobenzylidene malononitrile (CS) aerosol in three species of laboratory animal. Arch Toxicol, 52, 183–198.
13. Marrs TC, Clifford E and Colgrave HF (1983) Late inhalation toxicology and pathology produced by exposure to a single dose of 2-chlorobenzylidene malononitrile (CS) in rat and hamsters. Med Sci Law, 23, 257–265.
14. Upshall DG (1973) Effects of o-chlorobenzylidene malononitrile (CS) and the stress of aerosol inhalation upon rat and rabbit embryonic development. Toxicol Appl Pharmacol, 24, 45–59.
15. von Däniken A, Friederich U, Lutz WK and Schlatter C (1982) Tests for mutagenicity in Salmonella and covalent binding to DNA and protein in the rat of the riot control agent o-chlorobenzilidene malononitrile (CS). Arch Toxicol, 49, 15–27.
16. Meshram GP, Malini RP and Rao KM (1992) Mutagenicity evaluation of the riot control agent o-chlorobenzilidene malononitrile (CS) in the Ames Salmonella/microsome test. J Appl Toxicol, 12, 377–384.
17. McGregor DB, Brown A, Cattanach P et al. (1988) Responses of the L5178Y tk+/tk− mouse lymphoma cell forward mutation assay II: 18 coded chemicals. Environ Mol Mutagen, 11, 91–118.
18. Schmid E, Bauchinger M, Ziegler-Skylakakis K and Andrae U (1989) 2-Chlorobenzylidene malononitrile (CS) causes spindle disturbances in V79 Chinese hamster cells. Mutat Res, 226, 133–136.
19. Wild D, Eckhardt K, Harnasch D and King M-T (1983) Genotoxicity study of CS (ortho-chlorobenzylidene malononitrile in Salmonella, Drosophila and mice. Arch Toxicol, 54, 167–170.
20. Chowdhury AR, Rastogy VK, Arora U and Saxena C (1985) Biochemical and

morphological alteration of adrenal under the exposure of ortho-chlorobenzylidene malononitrile. *Mikroskopie (Wien)*, **42**, 151–156.

21. Shmunes E and Taylor JS (1973) Industrial contact dermatitis effect of the riot control agent ortho-chlorobenzilidene malononitrile. *Arch Dermatol*, **107**, 212–216.

22. Fuchs T and Ippen H (1986) Kontaktallergie auf CN- and CS-Tränengas. *Dermatosen*, **34**, 12–14.

23. Owens EJ and Punte CL (1963) Human respiratory and ocular irritation studies utilizing *o*-chlorobenzilidene malononitrile aerosols. *Ind Hyg J*, **24**, 262–264.

24. Beswick FW, Holland P and Kemp KH (1972) Acute effects of exposure to orthochlorobenzylidene malononitrile. *Br J Indust Med*, **29**, 298–306.

25. Park S and Giammona ST (1972) Toxic effects of tear gas on an infant following prolonged exposure. *Am J Dis Child*, **123**, 245–246.

26. Lee BH, Knopp R and Richardson ML (1984) Treatment of exposure to chemical personal protection agents. *Ann Emerg Med*, **13**, 123–124.

27. Kok-van Aalphen CC, Visser R, van der Linden JW and Bol AH (1985) Protection of the police against tear gas with soft contact lenses. *Military Med*, **150**, 451–454.

28. Ballantyne B (1977) Riot control agents. In: *Medical Annual*, pp. 7–41. Bristol: John Wright.

29. McNamara BP, Vocci FJ and Owens EJ (1968) The toxicology of CN. Edgewood Arsenal Technical Report No. 4207, December 1968, Edgewood Arsenal, Maryland USA.

30. WHO (1970) *Health Aspects of Chemical and Biological Weapons*. Report of a World Health Organization Group of Consultants. Geneva: WHO.

Appendix 1

ABBREVIATIONS FOR SOME CHEMICAL WARFARE AGENTS

Agent	Standard abbreviation	Other abbreviations
Tabun	GA	
Sarin	GB*	
Soman	GD	Thickened soman—TGD or VR_{55}.
—	VX	V agents are sometimes referred to as A or F agents
—	VE	
—	GE	
—	GF	
Sulphur mustard	H	HD; HS; LOST; BB
Mustard/lewisite mixture	HL	
Nitrogen mustard	HN_1	
Nitrogen mustard	HN_2	
Nitrogen mustard	HN_3	
Sesqui mustard	Q	
Lewisite	L	M-1
Phosgene	CG	D-stoff
Hydrogen cyanide	AC	French 4
Cyanogen chloride	CK	
Phosgene oxime	CX	
'Tear gas'	CN	
'Tear gas'	CS†	
'Tear gas'	CR	
Bromacetone	BA	

(continued overleaf)

(*continued*)

Agent	Standard abbreviation	Other abbreviations
Diphenylchlorarsine	DA	Clark I
Adamsite	DM	
Diphenylcyanarsine	DC	CDA; Clark II
Ethyldichlorarsine ⎱ Methyldichlorarsine ⎰ Phenyldichlorarsine	The 'Dicks'	MD
Phenyl acetonitrile 30% ⎱ Phenyl bromoacetonitrile 70% ⎰	BBC	CA, Bromobenzylcyanide, Camite
3-Quinuclidinyl benzilate	BZ[§]	
Chloropicrin	PS	Klop
Diphosgene	DP	
Ethyliodoacetate	SK[‡]	KSK
Disulphur decafluoride	Z	

*Sarin was a code name suggested by Schrader as a derivation of Schrader, Ambros, Rüdriger and Van der linde, the workers who synthesized the compound.
[†]CS was chosen as Corson and Stoughton developed the compound.
[‡]SK was chosen as the early work was done at Imperial College, South Kensington, London.
[§]BZ (3-Quinuclidinyl benzilate) is sometimes confused with benactyzine.

Appendix 2

APPROXIMATE FIGURES FOR HUMAN TOXICITY OF SOME CW AGENTS

LCt_{50} and LD_{50} values unless otherwise stated.

GB   70–100 mg min m^{-3}
0.01 mg kg^{-1} IV
Near max. miosis at $Ct = 15$ mg min m^{-3}

GD   40–60 mg min m^{-3}
0.025 mg kg^{-1}, IV
1.2 mg kg^{-1}, per cut

GA   150 mg min m^{-3}
0.08 mg kg^{-1}, IV

GF   1.0–1.4 mg per person, IV

VX   0.007 mg kg^{-1}, IV
0.142 mg kg^{-1}, per cut
50 mg min m^{-3}, aerosol

H   1500 mg min m^{-3}, inhaled
100 mg kg^{-1}, per cut
0.2 mg kg^{-1}, IV

L   1200 mg min m^{-3}
      2.6 g per person fatal, per cut

CG   3200 mg m^{-3}, LC_{50} (Note the figure quoted here is an LC_{50} figure and not an LCt_{50} figure.)

AC   1000–2000 mg min m^{-3}
      Max tolerable level 22 mg m^{-3}

CX ICt_{100}: Eye effects 3 mg min m^{-3}

INDEX

Index compiled by Liza Weinkove